The Road to Healthy Living

The Road to Healthy Living

Sharon L. Cavusgil

Ann Arbor
THE UNIVERSITY OF MICHIGAN PRESS

ISBN 0-472-08294-9
Library of Congress Catalog Card No. 94-61574
Published in the United States of America by
The University of Michigan Press
Manufactured in the United States of America

1998 1997 1996 1995 4 3 2 1

Series Introduction

Content-based instruction (CBI) is the integration of content and language learning. **Alliance: The Michigan State University Textbook Series of Theme-Based Content Instruction for ESL/EFL** is designed principally for postsecondary programs in English as a second/foreign language, though some books are appropriate for secondary programs as well. **Alliance** is the first series to allow programs to experiment with content-based language instruction without the demand of teachers' time and effort in developing materials. It also offers a wide selection of topics from which both teachers and students can choose.

The rationale for a content-based approach to language instruction comes from the claim that interesting and relevant material increases motivation and promotes effective language learning. CBI also adheres to the pedagogical principle that teaching should build on the previous subject matter *and* second language knowledge of the learner, while taking into account the eventual uses the learners will make of the second or foreign language. Finally, with a content-based approach, students will grow in not one but three areas: second-language acquisition, content knowledge, and cognitive development.

Three models of CBI at the postsecondary levels exist: theme-based, sheltered, and adjunct courses. The **Alliance** series utilizes a theme-based approach in which language skills, grammar, vocabulary, and cognitive skills are integrated into the study of one particular subject area. This model is advantageous in that it can be implemented in any postsecondary program and can be taught at all proficiency levels. Sheltered and adjunct courses, on the other hand, are limited to university settings with high-intermediate to advanced-level students. The theme-based approach is also preferable for this series as it is the only approach that has as its principal goal the improvement of language competence rather than mastery of subject material.

Unique Features of the Series

All the textbooks have been piloted in the classroom by teachers other than the author. Because content-based instruction is a relatively new area of language teaching, our goal is to produce textbooks that are accessible to those teachers who have a great deal of experience with CBI and to those who have little or no experience. By piloting the textbooks with different teachers, we confirmed that people unfamiliar with the topic were able to teach the material easily. One teacher who taught the ecology text said, "I am an English teacher and I know next to nothing about the topic of ecology. As it turned out, the book gave me all the information that I needed." This piloting also allowed the author to receive feedback on which activities worked and which didn't work, to determine whether or not the material was appropriate for the level and to check for any "loopholes" in the textbook.

The teacher's manual provides detailed explanations for those who may want more guidance for teaching the course. Detailed explanations and information for teaching the materials are in the teacher's manuals. Teachers can use or not use the information, depending on their experience, needs, and desires.

Each chapter in the student books states the content objectives, while teachers are provided with both content and language objectives in the teacher's manual. We expect that there is a range in teachers' philosophies toward CBI. Some teachers may accept wholly the idea that there should be no overt instruction of language and that students will naturally acquire the language through the content. Some, however, may feel that overt language instruction is necessary. By restricting the language objectives to the teacher's manual, teachers have the option to share them with their students or use them only as information to guide their teaching. The omission of the language objectives from the student's book also allows teachers to further develop any material and not feel obligated to cover "specified" language objectives.

Explanations of language items are clearly shown in "language boxes." Any detailed language point is explained in "language boxes." These boxes give teachers the option to cover the material in class or to leave the information as reference for students to use on their own, depending on their philosophy toward CBI. The information in the language boxes also saves valuable time since teachers do not have to find the supporting language explanations from other textbooks.

Each book is devoted entirely to one particular content that builds on the students' previous learning experiences. This type of in-depth coverage allows topic related vocabulary and concepts to be continuously recycled, thus increasing the students' knowledge of the content and language. Students will benefit from the coherence provided by an integrated skills approach with one unifying topical content.

The interest and needs of the learners are considered in the choice of topics. Our experience has shown that students have a wide variety of interests, some enjoying courses that are "entertainment" focused, such as music or film, while others prefer a more "academic" focus, such as American government or media. We have developed books that present different choices and are immediately relevant to and usable in a student's daily life.

Several choices of topics exist for the beginner, intermediate, and advanced level. As the student population varies from term to term, so will their needs and interests. Having more than one book to choose from at each level lets students choose the topics of special interest to them. Teachers can also choose topics they are comfortable with or interested in teaching.

Authentic materials are used whenever possible. One of the goals of CBI is to use original text that was created for a purpose other than language teaching. The structure, function, and discourse features in these materials then dictate what language is to be taught. While much of the information was kept in its original form, some of the authentic texts were adapted to match the language ability of the audience.

Content material is supplemented with activities that assist students in comprehension. The material in each book has been carefully analyzed to determine those language skills that will assist the students in comprehending the information. Activities have then been developed, and any necessary language explanations to accomplish this goal have been included.

Language items are presented in an inductive format. This format encourages students to generate themselves how or why a particular form is used. This "active" discovery helps students retain the information more successfully.

Format of the Books

Each book in the **Alliance** series follows the same format except in the Vocabulary Development section, present in some books but not in others. This format is as follows.

Opening Activity. Each chapter opens with some sort of activity that will get the students thinking about the topic of the chapter. This opening activity may be as simple as a picture or may involve a detailed activity. Its purpose is not to master the content described but simply to raise the students' awareness of the topic.

A Look Behind/A Look Ahead. This section contains a brief review of the previous chapter and an overview of what the students will study in the current chapter.

To the Student. Each chapter lists the content objectives, and students are encouraged to read these before studying the chapter as a preview. They should also go over the objectives again at the end of the chapter to check for comprehension.

Vocabulary Development. Some of the texts include a section on vocabulary development so that the students can have a list of important vocabulary words as well as to learn various strategies for developing that vocabulary.

Content Headings. The chapter is then divided into content areas marked with roman numerals. Within that content area, activities (labeled A, B, C, etc.) help students comprehend the material.

Series Acknowledgments

There are many people we need to thank for their help in making this series a reality. Most important, the authors deserve our gratitude for their dedication, insight, and cooperation toward the project despite their busy professional demands. We are also indebted to the entire staff at the English Language Center. Whether or not they were directly involved, everyone was willing to adjust schedules to accommodate and support the needs of the project. From our original meeting, Mary Erwin, our project editor at the University of Michigan Press, has been our major supporter, urging, pushing, and cajoling us to meet deadlines. Her belief in this project has ultimately allowed these materials to see the light of day. Special thanks also goes to Peter Shaw of the Monterey Institute, who initially envisioned this project.

We are aware that there are still many theoretical and practical issues left to be resolved surrounding content-based instruction. We hope the

Alliance series will make some inroads toward the resolution of some of the issues and lead to a better acceptance of this approach to language teaching in the field of ESL/EFL.

Susan Gass—Project Coordinator
Amy Tickle—Series Editor

Author's Acknowledgments

Several people deserve special thanks for their assistance with this text. I want to thank Sue Gass and Amy Tickle for their support, encouragement, and invaluable advice. Amy's thoughtful insight, suggestions, and humor got me through several bouts of writer's block. Others deserve a thank you—Kevin Burkitt and Freya Kakowski for piloting my text in their classrooms and U of M Press reviewers for reviewing the text and providing helpful suggestions for revision. Lastly, I want to thank my husband Alper, who patiently listened to my ideas and frustrations. Without his support, I could not have completed this text. I look forward to comments from teachers and students who use this text.

Sharon L. Cavusgil

To the Student

Good health is very important. Good health includes a healthy mind and a healthy body. It means proper food, exercise, and relaxation. This book will help you develop a healthy attitude and lifestyle. It also will help you adapt to a new culture and customs. You will learn about different health scenarios at school, work, or home. And each chapter will help you improve your English skills.

Congratulations! You are moving in the right direction—toward a healthier lifestyle!

Contents

Introduction

A. The following pictures introduce you to this textbook. First, study the pictures and talk about them. Who are these people? Where are they? Have you been in these situations?

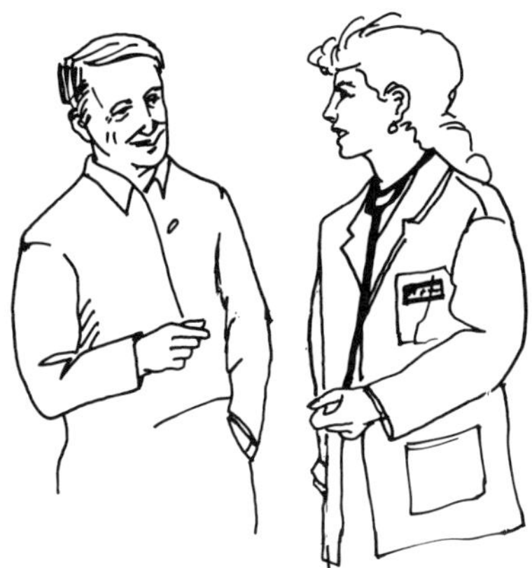

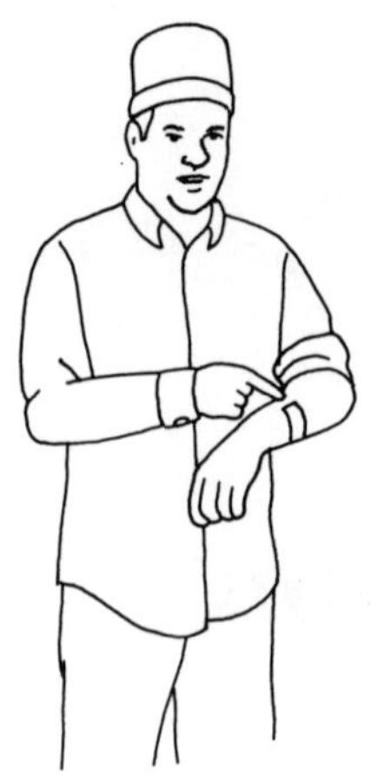

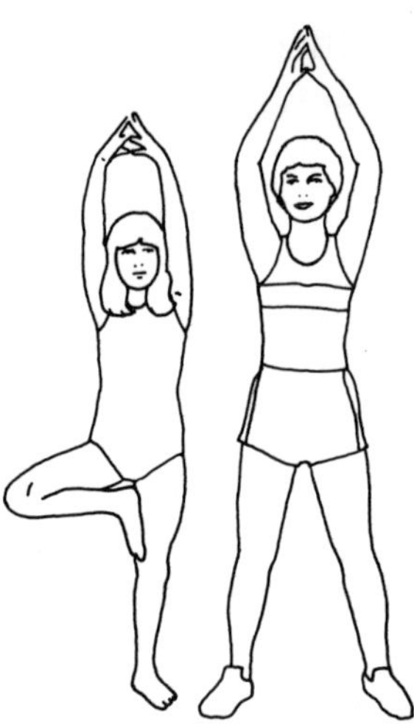

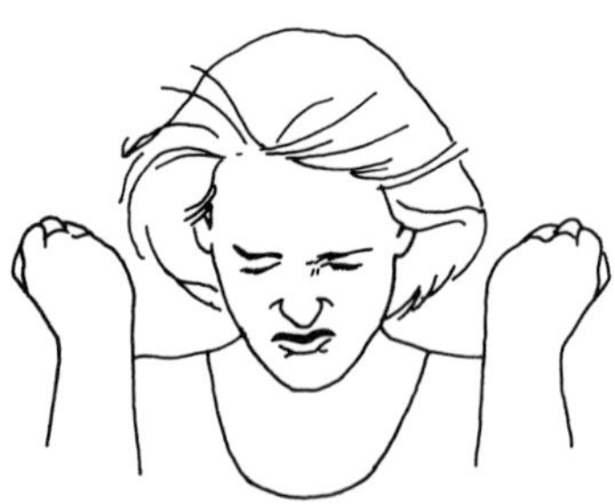

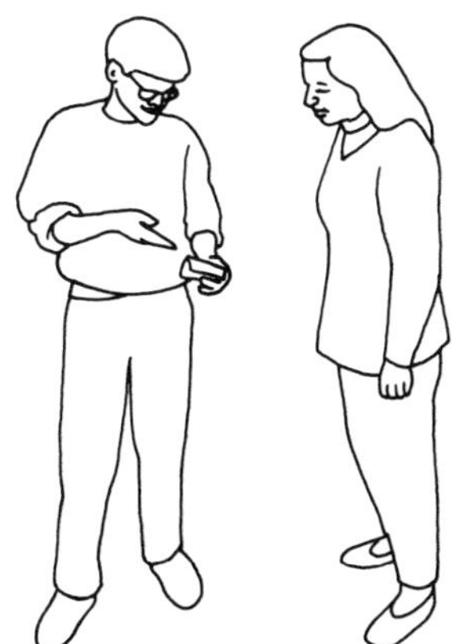

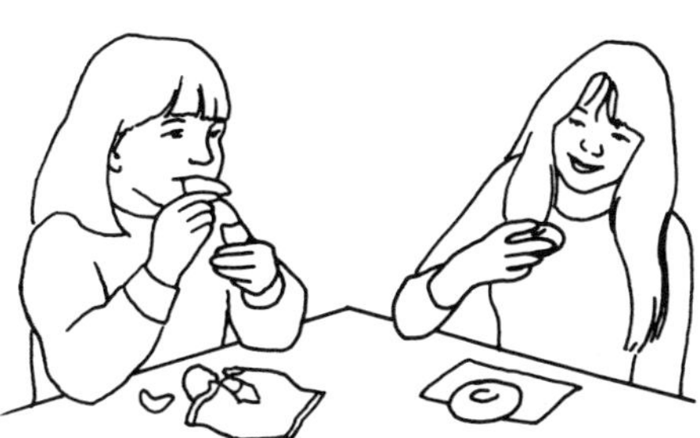

B. Now, find the sentence about each picture. Write the sentence on the line below the correct picture.

1. Manuel talks with his doctor.
2. Sharon and Jigna exercise at the center.
3. Pablo explains a label.
4. Ahmed describes his illness.
5. Berin and Margareta eat junk food.
6. Marissa is stressed.

Chapter 1

The Human Body

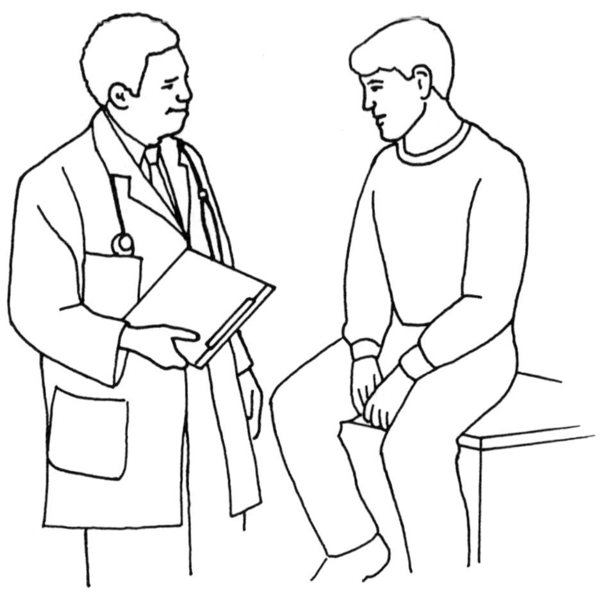

A Look Ahead

When you are sick in a new culture, it is frightening. It is also stressful. Your health is important. You need to make good decisions. Should you see a doctor? Should you take medicine? Can you explain your illness? You must be confident with your English. This book brings you closer to good health.

In this chapter, you will learn the English words for the parts of the human body.

To the Student

After completing this chapter, you will be able to

1. use the vocabulary of the human body parts.

Vocabulary Development

In English, all words have one or more syllables. A syllable is a word part that has a vowel sound. A dictionary shows the syllables in a word. It uses a dot (·) or a hyphen (-).

Examples:

head /hɛd/ *n* the part of the body that contains the eyes, nose, mouth, and ears

el·bow /'ɛlbo^{w} / *n* the place where the arm bends

Head has one syllable, and *elbow* has two syllables. You can learn to say a new word by pronouncing one syllable at a time.

The following are some important words from chapter 1. Use your dictionary to mark the syllables in each word. For words with only one syllable, do nothing. The first three words are done for you.

___ ankle an·kle	___ wrist ______	___ back ______
___ chin chin	___ eyebrow ______	___ chest ______
___ finger fin·ger	___ nose ______	___ elbow ______
___ forehead ______	___ head ______	___ heel ______
___ stomach ______	___ tooth ______	___ shin ______
___ knee ______	___ mouth ______	___ shoulder ______
___ muscle ______	___ bone ______	___ heart ______
___ kidney ______	___ brain ______	___ lung ______
___ vein ______	___ throat ______	___ nerve ______
______	______	______
______	______	______

Now, let's focus on the meaning of these words. Read the list again. If you already understand the word, put a check (✓) on the line to the left of the word. When you finish this chapter, return to this list again. Check off all the new words you learned. Write in additional words you have learned that are not on the list, too. You will use these words again, so review them often.

I. From Head to Toe

A. To communicate your illnesses, you need to know vocabulary for the parts of your body. Label the body parts you already know. Ask a classmate to help you with the other body parts.

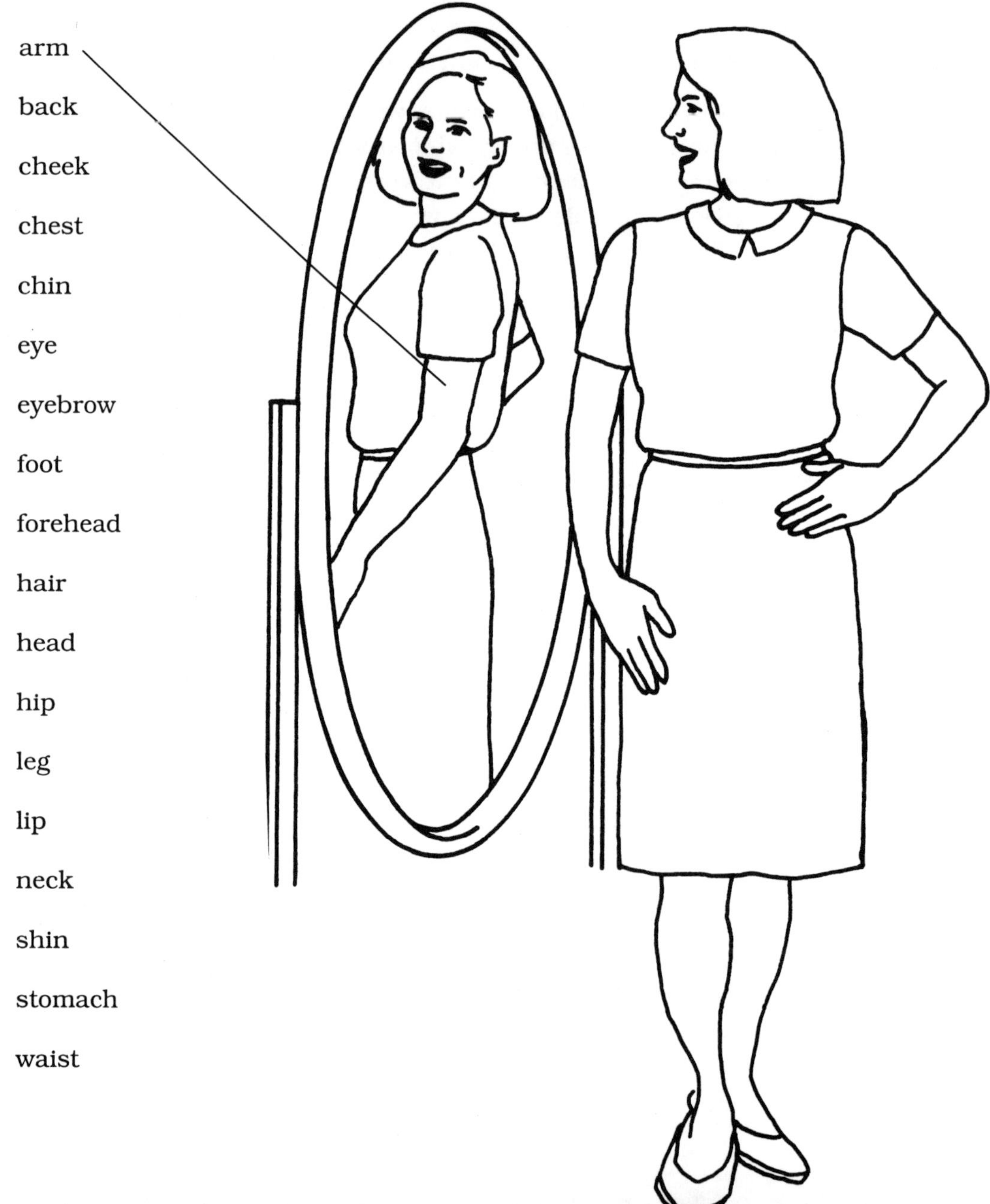

B. Start at the top of the body, and pronounce each word after your teacher. Your teacher may ask, "What's *this* called?" You should respond, "*That* is a (an) ____________." For example,

What is this?

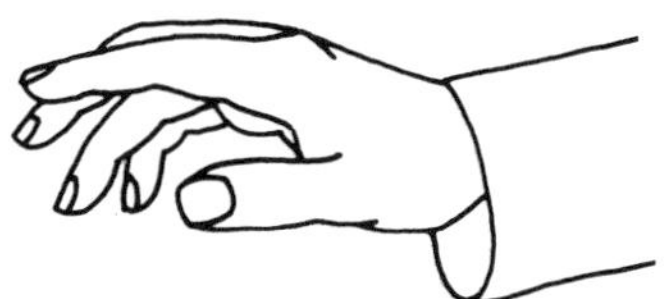

That's a hand.

What are these?

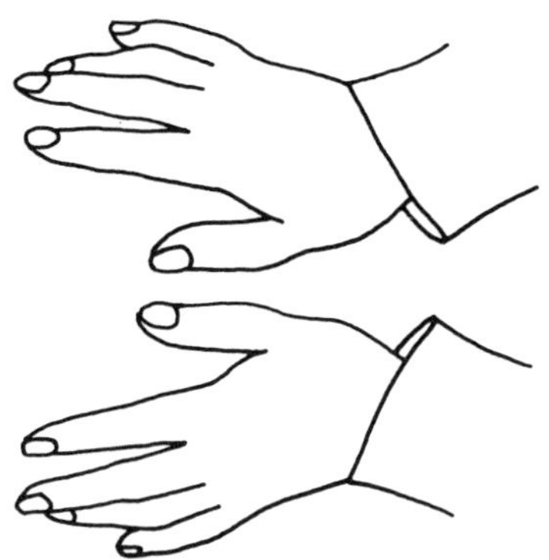

Those are hands.

Demonstratives: *This, That, These,* and *Those*

Singular	*Plural*	*Usage*
this	*these*	the object(s) are near you
that	*those*	the object(s) are not near you

The Verb *Be: Is* and *Are*

Singular			*Plural*		
This	*is*	my nose.	These	*are*	my eyes.
That	*is*	your head.	Those	*are*	his arms.
The doctor	*is*	at the hospital.	The nurses	*are*	at the hospital.
The book	*is*	on my desk.	The books	*are*	on my desk.
It	*is*	on my desk.	They	*are*	on my desk.

C. Follow the pattern your teacher used. Work with a partner and practice using the body parts vocabulary. One student points to a body part (or parts) and asks a question. The other student gives the correct response. Be sure to use the correct demonstrative and form of the verb *be.*

D. The human body has main body parts. For example, the hand is a main body part. The thumb and fingers belong to the hand. One word in each of the following groups does not belong to the body part. Cross out the word that does not belong. If you do not know a word, use your dictionary.

Example:

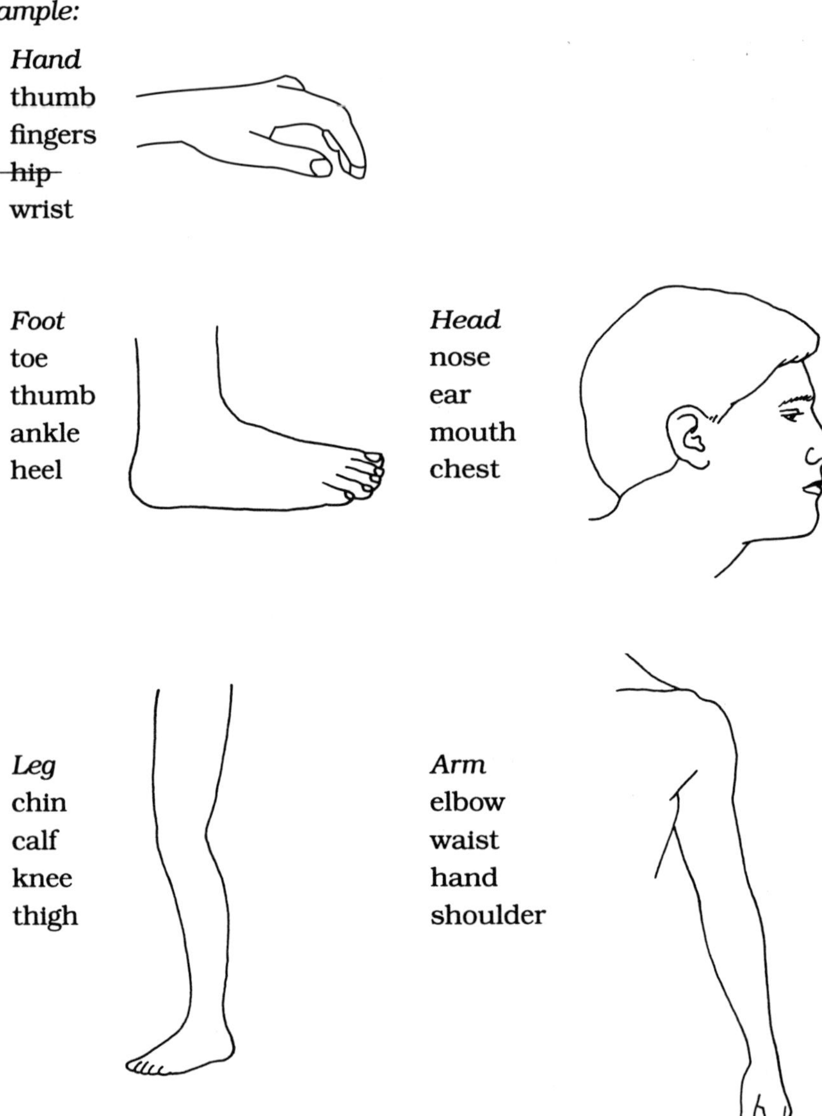

Hand
thumb
fingers
~~hip~~
wrist

Foot
toe
thumb
ankle
heel

Head
nose
ear
mouth
chest

Leg
chin
calf
knee
thigh

Arm
elbow
waist
hand
shoulder

E. The following sentences use the prepositions *above* and *below.*

Examples:

The nose is above the chin and below the forehead.

The eyes are above the mouth and below the eyebrows.

Prepositions of Location: *Above* and *Below*

Prepositions sometimes describe the location of things. Two common prepositions of location are *above* and *below.*

An airplane can fly *above* the clouds.

On a map, Mexico lies *below* the United States.

Look at the prepositions in the following sentences. Complete each sentence with an appropriate body part.

1. The ______________ is above the foot and below the thigh.
2. The ______________ is above the hips and below the chest.
3. The neck is above the ______________ and below the ______________.
4. The knee is above the ______________ and below the ______________.

Now, write your own sentences.

5. ______________
6. ______________
7. ______________
8. ______________

II. Inside and Out

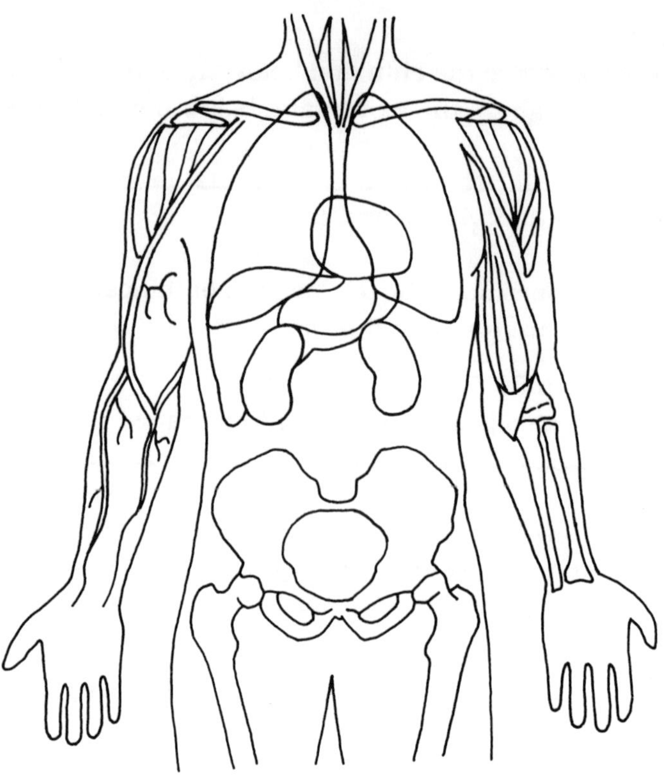

A. It is also important to know the terms for the parts inside your body (internal body parts). Study the human diagram. How many internal body parts do you know? To help you learn these words, write the list of internal body parts in alphabetical order next to the numbers. Then, use a dictionary to write the definition of each word. The first two words are defined for you.

kidney	muscle	heart	lung	throat
stomach	nerve	brain	bone	vein

1. bone—the hard parts of the body that support the body and protect the organs
2. brain—the organ in the head that controls actions, thoughts, and feelings
3. heart—______________________________________
4. ____

5. ______________________________

6. ______________________________

7. ______________________________

8. ______________________________

9. ______________________________

10. ______________________________

B. Use your definitions and match the internal body part to the appropriate function.

Internal Body Part	*Function of Body Part*
1. _______ heart	a. is inside the neck area
2. _______ lung	b. controls actions, thoughts, and feelings
3. _______ kidney	c. carries blood to other body parts
4. _______ muscle	d. digests food
5. _______ vein	e. cleans the blood
6. _______ nerve	f. supports and protects internal organs
7. _______ brain	g. tightens to produce movement
8. _______ bone	h. carries messages to and from the brain
9. _______ stomach	i. breathes air
10. _______ throat	j. pumps blood throughout the body

III. Parts and More Parts

A. Some parts of the body are plural. For example, you have two legs, two ears, and two arms. Most of these words form their plural by adding -s. These plural words have different pronunciations. Look at the following three words:

nerves
thighs
noses

Pronounce these words aloud and listen to their plural endings. What do they sound like?

Pronunciation of -*s* Endings

In English there are three pronunciations of the -*s* ending.

When a word ends in the consonants /p/, /t/, /f/, /k/, and /θ/ (*th* as in *thin* or *through*), pronounce the plural ending like the *s* in *sad.*

body part → body parts
lip → lips

When a word ends in the consonants /b/, /d/, /g/, /v/, /m/, /n/, /ŋ/ (*ng* as in *thing*), /l/, /r/, and /ð/ (*th* as in *this* or *though*), pronounce the plural ending like the *z* in *zero.*

leg → legs
doctor → doctors

When a word ends in a vowel or a vowel sound, also pronounce the plural ending like the *z* in *zero.*

toe → toes
thigh → thighs

When a word ends in the sounds /s/ or /z/, or the letters *j, sh,* and *ch,* pronounce the plural ending as /ɪz/. The plural is pronounced as a separate syllable.

face → fac-es
nose → nos-es

B. Pronounce the following words and draw a line to connect each word to the appropriate plural ending sound. For example, *bones* ends in a *z* sound.

bones	s
faces	
ankles	z
eyes	
cheeks	ɪz

C. Columns for the three plural -*s* endings follow. Listen to the dictation of the plural body parts vocabulary. You will hear each word twice. After the second time, pronounce the word aloud to yourself. Determine the plural ending sound and write the body part under the appropriate column. An example is provided.

/s/	/z/	/ɪz/
	eyes	

D. For each item, listen to the speaker pronounce four words. These words will be pronounced twice. Concentrate on the sound of the plural ending of each word (s, z, or ɪz). Circle the word that ends in a different plural sound.

Example: ears elbows (cheeks) shins

1. hips thighs thumbs eyes
2. legs knees ankles noses
3. eyebrows lips fingers heels
4. shoulders arms wrists hands
5. muscles stomachs hearts throats

Some nouns do not add *-s* to form their plural. These nouns are irregular plural nouns.

Irregular Plural Nouns

Singular Nouns	*Irregular Plural Nouns*
foot	feet
tooth	teeth

E. List all the irregular plural nouns you can think of.

Chapter 2

Health Problems and Their Symptoms

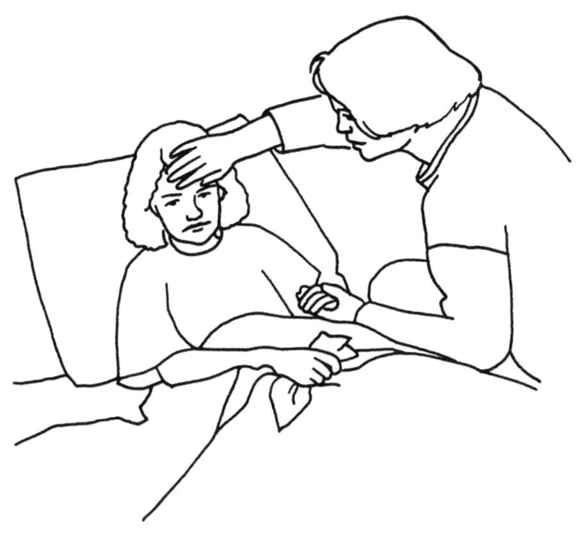

A Look Behind/A Look Ahead

In chapter 1, you learned the parts of the human body. This knowledge can help you describe your illnesses. In a new environment, you can easily get sick. You are busy at school or with work. You meet many new people. You have many changes in your life. With all of this, you might not take good care of yourself. Can you explain to a friend, a teacher, an employer, or a doctor how you are feeling? Can you confidently do this in English? Chapter 2 helps you describe your health problems and explain their symptoms.

To the Student

After completing this chapter, you will be able to

1. describe health problems and their symptoms;
2. respond to greetings at school, work, or social events; and
3. cancel plans or "call in" sick to work or school because of an illness.

Vocabulary Development

In chapter 1, you studied syllables. You can learn to say a new word by pronouncing one syllable at a time. In addition, it is important to understand which syllable to say with more force (stress). A dictionary shows stress in a word. It uses a mark (').

Examples:

head·ache /'hɛdek/ *n* a pain in the head
fe·ver /'fivər/ *n* an illness; a high body temperature
de·vel·op /dɪ'vɛləp/ *v* to grow, increase

In *headache* and *fever,* the stress is on the first syllable. In *develop,* the stress is on the second syllable.

The following are some of the important words or phrases from chapter 2. Use your dictionary to mark the syllables and stress in each word. For words with only one syllable, do nothing. The first three words are done for you.

__ cough <u>cough</u>	__ symptom ______	__ sore ______
__ headache <u>'head·ache</u>	__ sick ______	__ rash ______
__ greet <u>greet</u>	__ the flu ______	__ illness ______
__ hurt ______	__ a cold ______	__ fever ______
__ toothache ______	__ ache ______	__ pain ______
______	______	______

______________________ ______________________ ______________________

______________________ ______________________ ______________________

______________________ ______________________ ______________________

Now, let's focus on the meaning of these words. Read the list again. If you already understand the word, put a check (✓) on the line to the left of the word. When you finish this chapter, return to the list. Check all new words you learned. Write in additional words you have learned that are not on the list, too. You will use these words again, so review them often.

I. What's the Matter?

A. Look at the pictures. What is wrong with these people? Fill in the missing words.

What's wrong?

Example

My __back__ hurts.
I have a sore __back__.

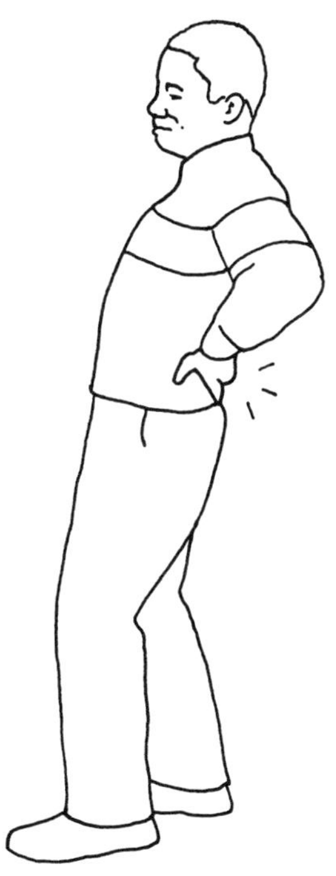

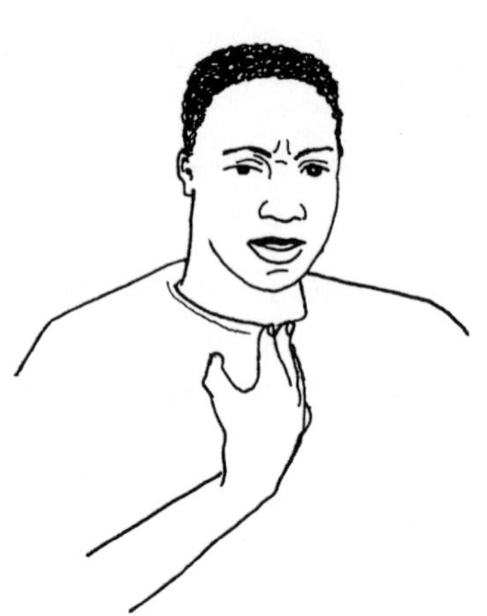

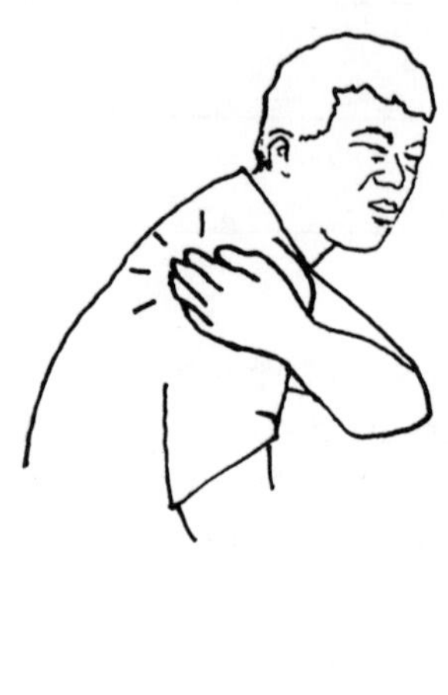

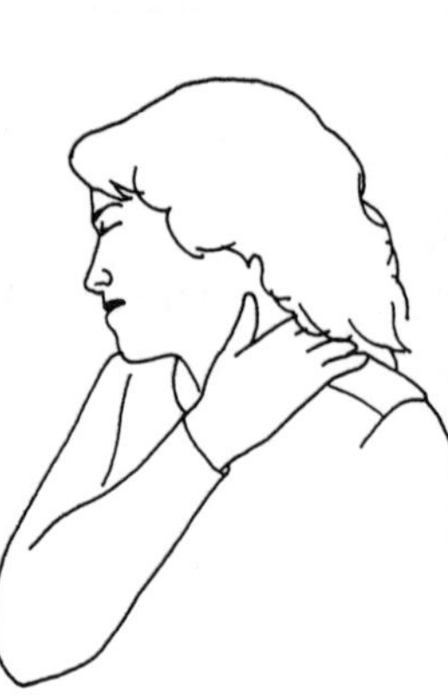

1. His ____________________ hurts.

   He has a sore _______________.

3. Their ____________________.

   They have _______________.

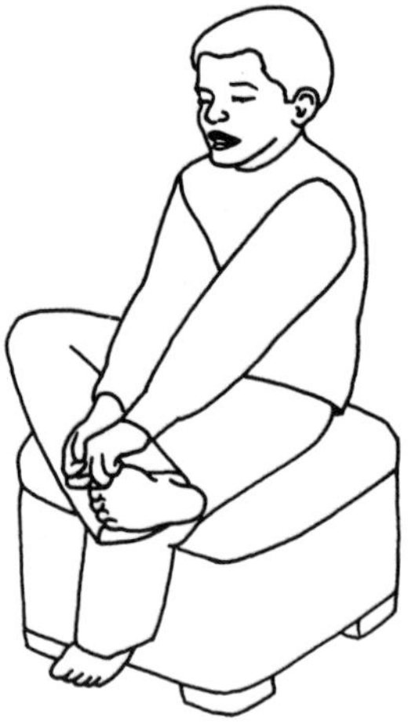

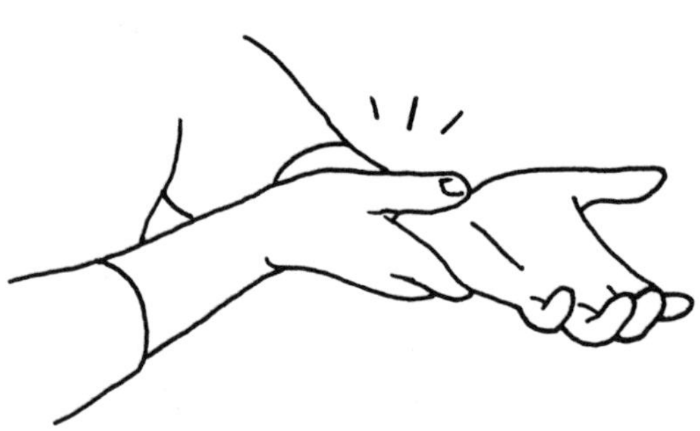

2. Your ____________________ hurts.

   You have a sore _______________.

4. Her ____________________.

   She has _______________.

The Present Tense of the Verb *Have: Has* and *Have*

The form of the verb *have* must agree with the subject. The singular form can be *has* or *have*. The plural form is *have*.

	Singular			*Plural*	
I	*have*	a headache.	We	*have*	sore feet.
You	*have*	an earache.	You	*have*	stomachaches.
Sharon	*has*	a sore arm.	The girls	*have*	sore throats.
She	*has*	a sore arm.	They	*have*	sore throats.
Michael	*has*	a toothache.	The boys	*have*	backaches.
He	*has*	a toothache.	They	*have*	backaches.
The dog	*has*	a sore tail.	The dogs	*have*	sore tails.
It	*has*	a sore tail.	They	*have*	sore tails.

B. Look at the additional pictures. What is wrong with these people? Fill in the missing words. Be sure to use the correct form of the verb *have*.

What's the matter?

Example
My __head__ hurts.
I have a __headache__.

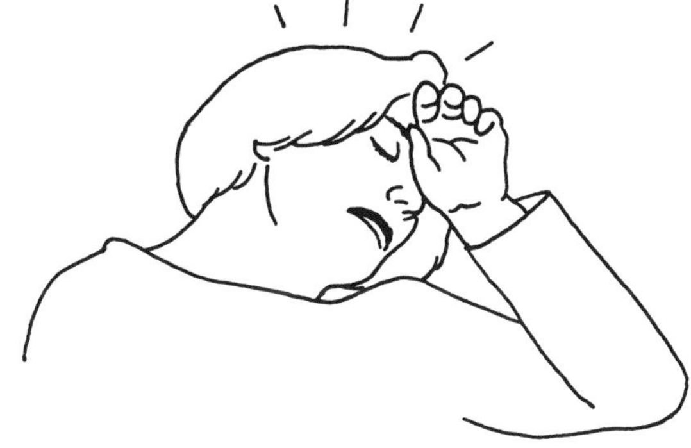

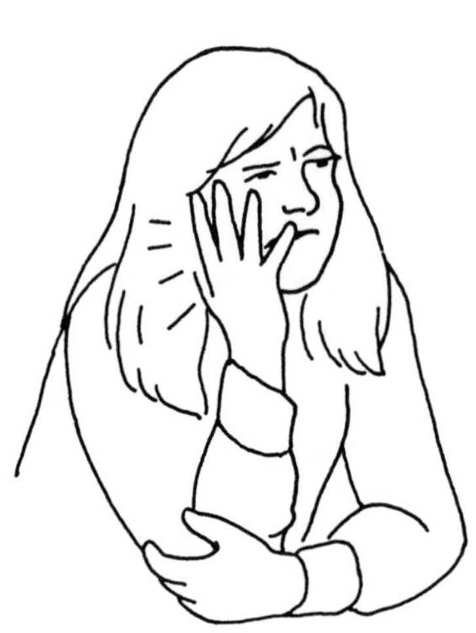

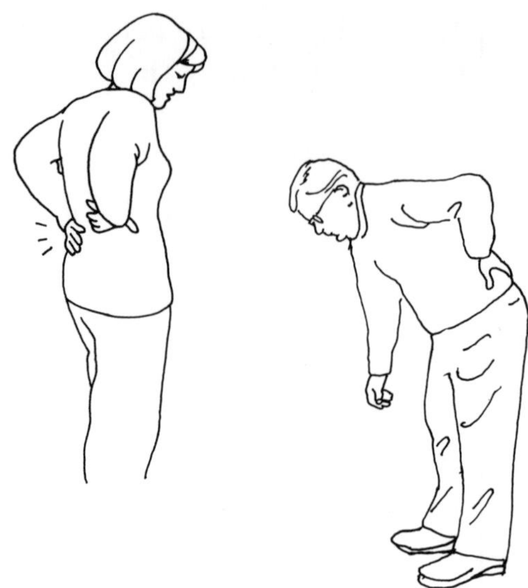

1. Her ________________ hurts.

   She has ________________.

3. Their ________________.

   They ________________.

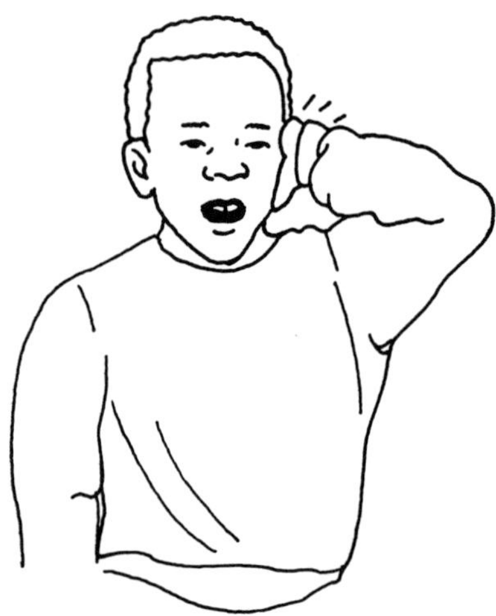

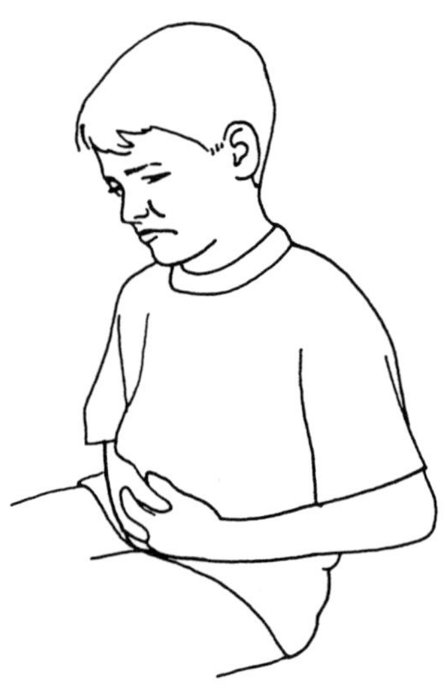

2. My ________________ hurts.

   I ________________.

4. Your ________________.

   You ________________.

C. Study each picture and then read the descriptions. Match a description to the appropriate picture and write it on the line.

I have a rash.	She has a cough.
Susan has a fever.	I have the flu.
He has a runny nose.	Robert has a cold.

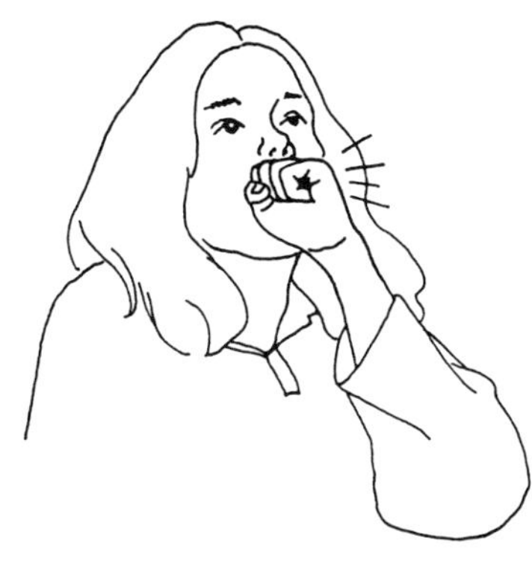

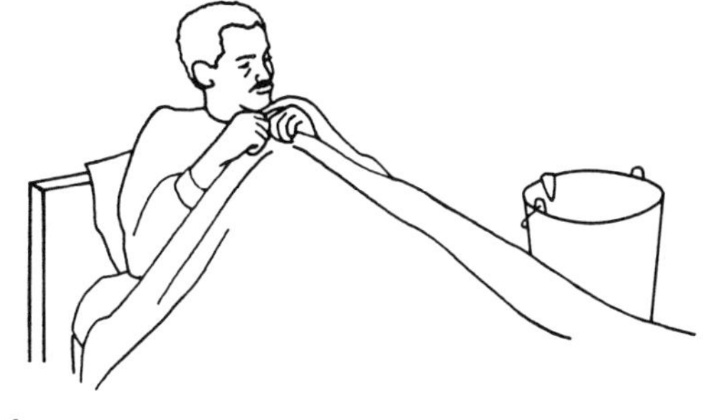

1. ____________________ 4. ____________________

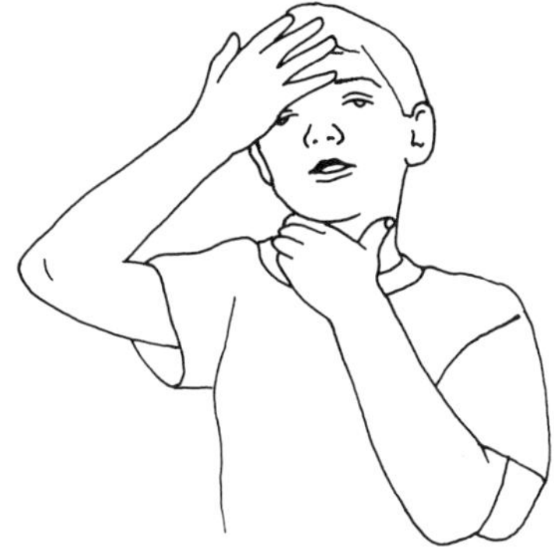

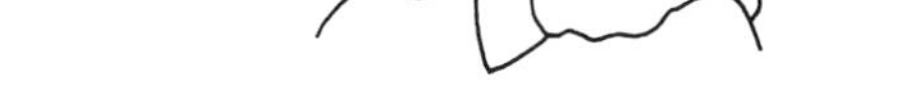

2. ____________________ 5. ____________________

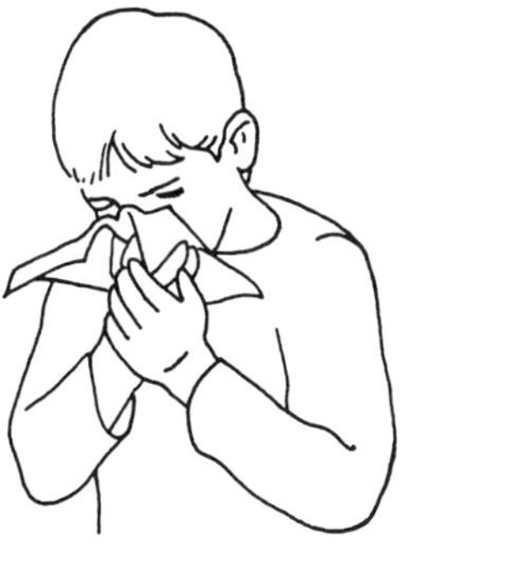

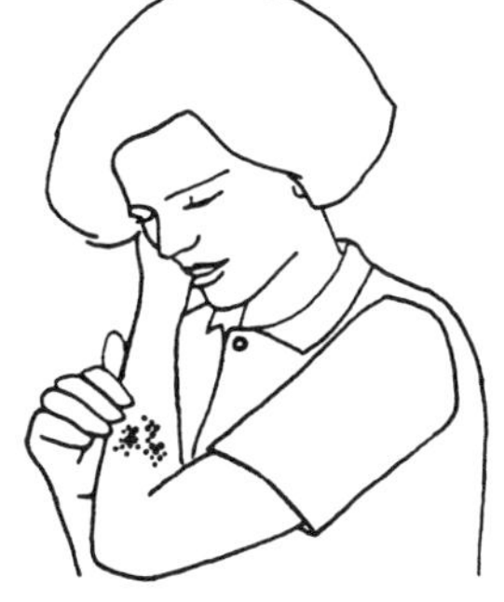

3. ____________________ 6. ____________________

D. When you visit the doctor, you may need to explain the symptoms of your illness. A symptom is something you feel or see when you are sick. For example, with a cough, your symptoms are an itchy, sore throat. Read the following symptoms. Which illness from Activity C *best* explains these symptoms?

Symptoms	*Illness*
1. red, itchy, sore skin	______________
2. hot and sore body, chills, vomiting	______________
3. headache, sore throat, runny nose, cough	______________
4. high temperature	______________
5. red, sore nose	______________

E. Turn to the Introduction on pages 1–3. Study the sentences for each picture. Identify the subjects, verbs, and objects. If the sentence part is made up of more than one word, draw a line under the entire sentence part. The first sentence is done for you.

1. Manuel (S) talks with (V) his doctor (O).
2. Sharon and Jigna exercise at the center.
3. Pablo explains a label.
4. Ahmed describes his illness.
5. Berin and Margareta eat junk food.
6. Marissa is stressed.

Basic Sentence Structure

The parts of a sentence include subjects, verbs, and objects. The sentence structure is subject + verb (+ object). Every sentence has a subject and a verb. Every sentence does not have an object.

Examples:

S V O
The boy hurt his finger.

S V
It is sore.

- A verb may describe an action (action verb). Or a verb may tell what something or someone is (being verb). *Hurt* is an action verb; *is* is a being verb.
- A subject is the thing or person that does the action. *The boy* and *it* are both subjects.
- An object is the thing or person that receives the action. In the first sentence, *his finger* is the object. There is no object in the second sentence.

F. In English, the simple present verb form is used for an action or a state of being that is true at the time of speaking. Study the verb forms in the following sentences. These are forms of the simple present tense.

I *see* a doctor once a year.	(first person singular)
You *see* a doctor once a year.	(second person singular)
She *sees* a doctor once a year.	(third person singular)
I *am* sick.	(first person singular)
You *are* sick.	(second person singular)
He *is* sick.	(third person singular)

Simple Present: *Be*

Singular			*Plural*		
I	*am*	sick.	We	*are*	sick.
You	*are*	sick.	You	*are*	sick.
He	*is*	sick.	They	*are*	sick.
She	*is*	sick.	They	*are*	sick.

Simple Present Verb Form

	Singular			*Plural*	
I	*visit*	the doctor.	We	*visit*	the doctor.
You	*visit*	the doctor.	You	*visit*	the doctor.
He	*visits*	the doctor.	They	*visit*	the doctor.
She	*visits*	the doctor.	They	*visit*	the doctor.

G. Complete the following sentences with the correct present form of the verb. Then, identify the sentence parts (S, V, O).

Example:

S V O

My roommate (eat) *eats* dinner early.

1. Rob (have) ____________________ a bad cold.

2. My mom and dad (call) ____________________ me every Saturday.

3. Donna (see) ____________________ her doctor once a year.

4. I (be) ____________________ very sick.

5. Those women (walk) ____________________ every morning.

6. I (love) ____________________ my family very much.

7. My friend (cook) ____________________ a healthy meal once a day.

8. Friday and Saturday (be) ____________________ my favorite days of the week.

II. My Head Hurts

A.

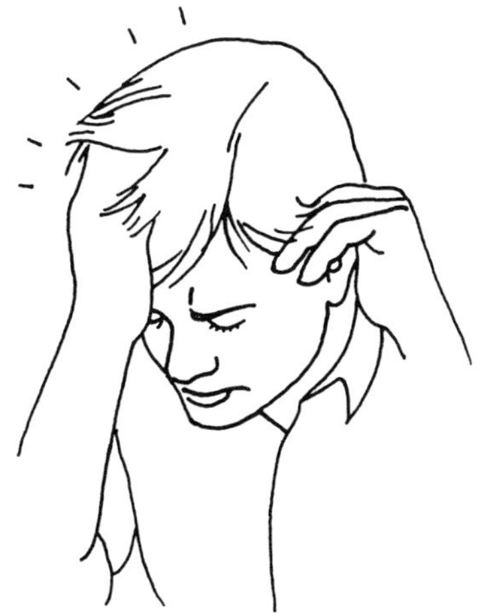

I have a headache.
My head hurts.

Pronoun Cases: Subjective, Objective, and Possessive

In the previous sentences, *I* and *my* are pronouns. English has three different pronoun cases.

> *I* have a sore throat.
> The doctor examines *me*.
> The doctor looks at *my* throat.

I is in the subjective case, *me* is in the objective case, and *my* is in the possessive case. We use the subjective and possessive cases to explain about body parts.

Subjective	*Objective*	*Possessive*
I	me	my, mine
you	you	your, yours
she	her	her, hers
he	him	his
it	it	its
we	us	our, ours
they	them	their, theirs

B. Look at the pictures. Complete each sentence to explain what is wrong with the people. First, use the appropriate subjective case. Then, use the possessive case to write additional sentences. To begin, study the example.

Subjective	*Possessive*

Example:

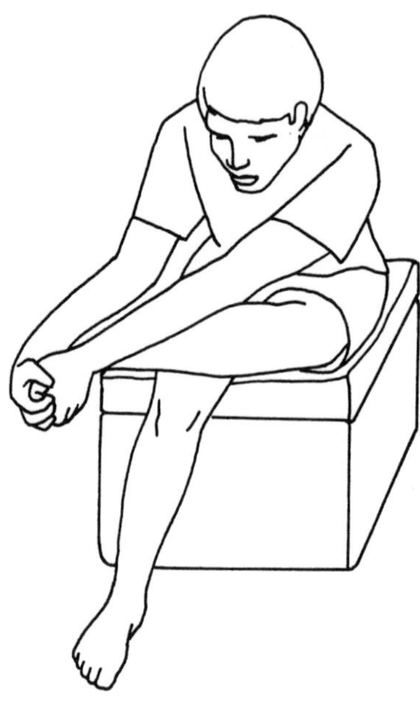

Subjective	Possessive
I have a sore foot.	*My* foot hurts.
	I hurt *my* foot.

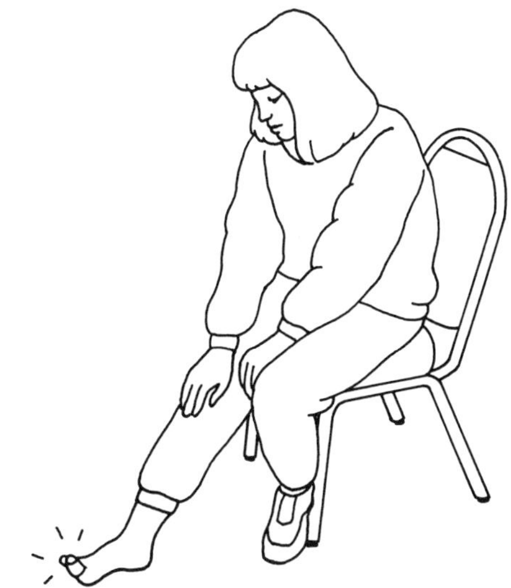

1. She has a ________________ Her ________________________

She hurt ____________________

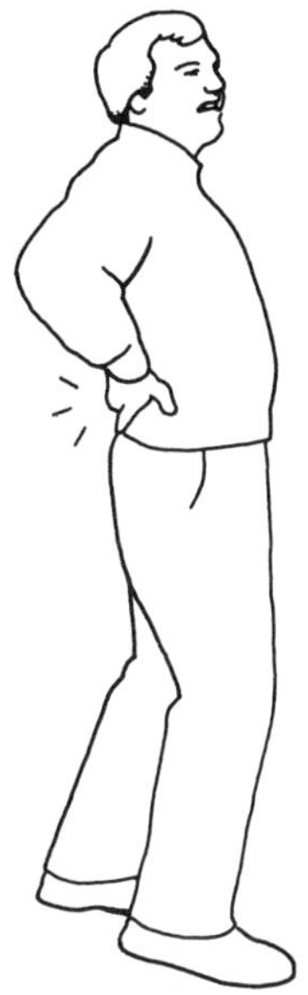

2. He has ________________ His ________________________

____

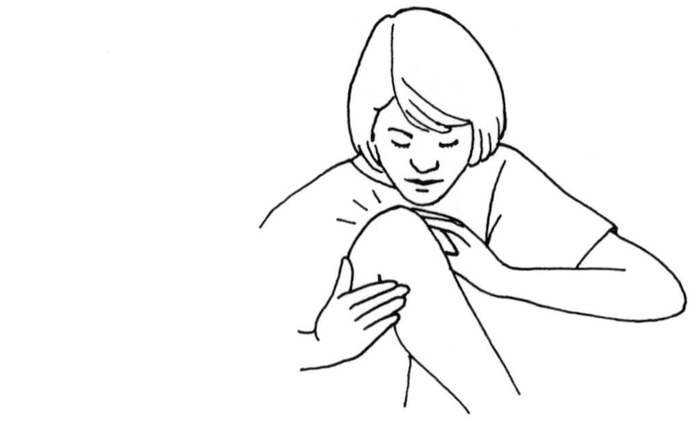

3. ______________________ Her ______________________

____

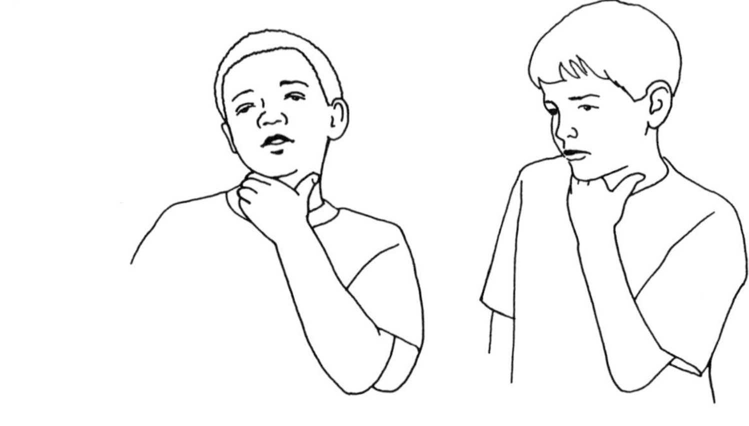

4. ______________________ ______________________

____

III. Hi! How Are You?

A. There are many different and correct ways to say hello to someone. A greeting can be casual or formal. Sometimes, the same greeting can be used in both casual and formal situations. Decide if the following greetings are casual (C), formal (F), or both (B). The first one is done for you.

1. Hi. ___C___
2. What's up? ______
3. Hello. ______
4. How are ya? ______
5. How ya doing? ______
6. Good morning. ______
7. How are you doing? ______
8. What's happening? ______
9. Hey! ______
10. How are you? ______

B. Decide how formal you should be with the following people. Write the person at the appropriate space on the line. An example is provided for you.

best friend	boss	classmate
neighbor	parent	young child
teacher	store clerk	bus driver

very casual — very formal

best friend ____

C. In the United States, a common greeting is "Hi. How are you?" Sometimes, the person is asking about your health. But usually the person is simply saying "hello." The person does not usually wish to hear about your health. An appropriate response is, "I'm fine. How are you?" With your classmates, discuss your experiences with this American greeting. When is it appropriate to give details about your health?

D. Study the pictures on page 30 and fill in the "bubbles" with appropriate greetings. Use greetings from Activity A.

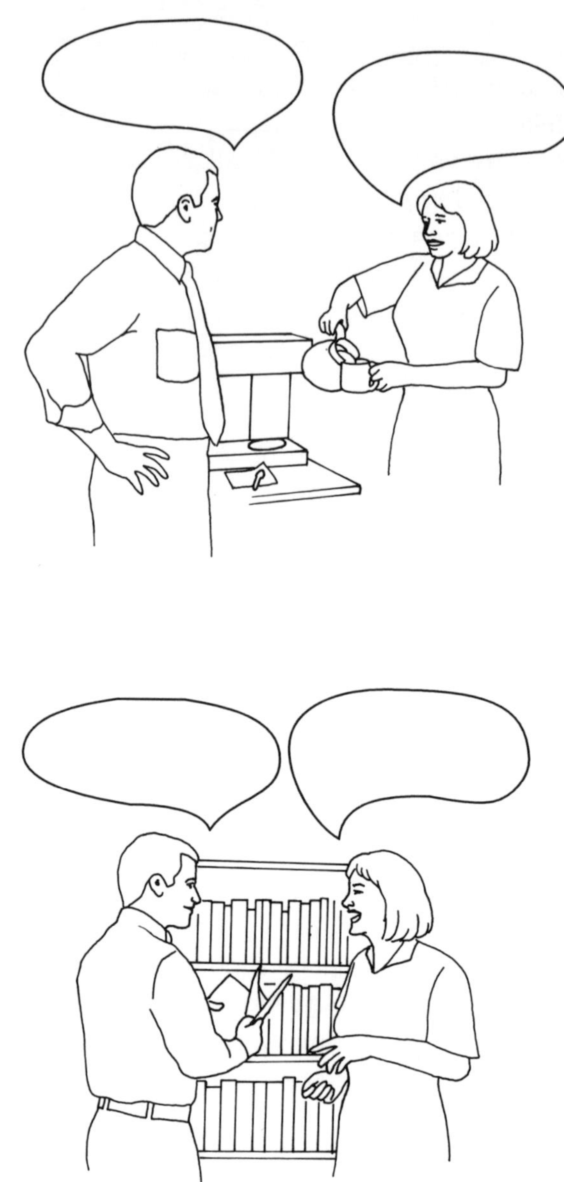

E. Go to a place where there are a lot of people (a cafeteria, the library, a store). Observe how people greet each other, and complete the chart as follows.

Verbal Greeting	Write the greeting (hello, how are you, etc.).
Body Greeting	Explain what the people do (shake hands, wave, nod their heads, smile, hug, etc.).
Formality	Decide on the greeting's level of formality (casual, formal, very formal).

Relationship Make a guess about the relationship of the people (friends, classmates, teacher/student, employee/employer, etc.).

Verbal Greeting	Body Greeting	Formality	Relationship

IV. "Calling In" Sick

Everyone gets sick. Sometimes, they don't go to school or work. Then, they call their employer or maybe their teacher. In addition, people sometimes don't feel well, so they cancel social plans. Certain language skills are used in these situations.

A. Listen to the two telephone conversations of Erin Larson.

Conversation A

Receptionist: Good morning, Bloomington Company.

Erin: May I speak to Ms. Wald, please.

Receptionist: One moment.

Ms. Wald: Ms. Wald speaking.

Erin: Ms. Wald, this is Erin Larson. I'm calling because I can't come in today. I have the flu.

Ms. Wald: Oh. I'm sorry to hear that, Erin. Thank you for calling. I hope you feel better soon. Call again tomorrow if you are still sick.

Erin: Yes, I will. Thank you.

Conversation B

Erin: Hi, Carlos. This is Erin. I'm sorry, but I can't go to the movies tonight. I don't feel well.

Carlos: Oh, what's wrong, Erin?

Erin: I think I have the flu. I have a headache and a fever. Also, my body aches all over.

Carlos: Ah, that's too bad. I hope you feel better. Is there anything I can do?

Erin: No, Carlos, but thanks for asking. Have fun at the movies, and let's get together soon!

Carlos: Okay! Take care, Erin.

B. Answer the following questions.

1. Who is Erin talking to (a friend, an employer, a teacher, etc.)?

   Conversation A ______________________________

   Conversation B ______________________________

2. In each conversation, when did Erin identify herself? Underline the sentences.

3. In each conversation, when did Erin give her reason for calling? Put two lines under the sentences.

4. In each conversation, when did Erin give her excuse? Circle the sentences.

5. How did Erin explain her illness (gave a lot of detail, gave a little detail)?

   Conversation A ______________________________

   Conversation B ______________________________

6. How did the conversation end (casually, formally)?

   Conversation A ______________________________

   Conversation B ______________________________

C. With a partner, select and write out the dialogue for one of the following situations. Be sure the dialogue is appropriate for each situation. Then, present your dialogue to the class. Have an appropriate apology, explanation, and excuse.

1. You have a sore throat. You tell a friend that you cannot come to his/her dinner party.
2. You have the flu. You explain to your boss why you want to leave work early.
3. You have a stomachache. You tell your teacher that you cannot take a test this afternoon.
4. Your tooth hurts. You inform your employer that you will not come to work today.
5. You have a skin rash. You tell a friend that you cannot babysit her/his daughter tomorrow.
6. You broke your leg. You explain to your teacher that you will be absent this week.

Chapter 3

Home Remedies

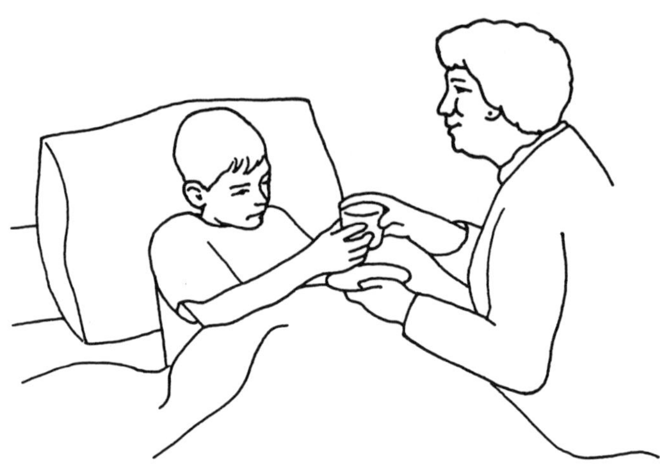

A Look Behind/A Look Ahead

In chapter 2, you learned how to describe your health problems and their symptoms. When people are sick, they try many things to feel better. Each culture has different customs and beliefs. For a fever, people from one country believe you should drink cold liquids. People from another country believe you should drink hot liquids. On the other hand, some home remedies (cures or suggestions) are universal. For example, most cultures believe that tea can relieve basic pains such as a sore throat.

In chapter 3, you will learn about your classmates' cultural home remedies and other suggestions for different health concerns.

To the Student

After completing this chapter, you will be able to

1. discuss home remedies for common illnesses, aches, and pains;
2. share remedies from your native country; and
3. give health advice.

Vocabulary Development

In chapters 1 and 2, you studied syllables and stress. A dictionary helps you understand syllables and stress. This helps you pronounce new words. A dictionary can also help you understand parts of speech (noun, verb, adjective, adverb, or preposition). In a dictionary, parts of speech are shown like this:

n = noun
v = verb
adj = adjective
adv = adverb
prep = preposition

Examples:

head·ache /'hɛdek/ ⓝ a pain in the head
greet /grit/ ⓥ to welcome in a friendly way

The following are some of the important words from chapter 3. Use your dictionary to mark the syllables and stress in each word. Then, write the part of speech on the line. The first three words are done for you.

n advice ad·'vice	___ remedy ______	___ cure ______
v expand ex·'pand	___ symptom ______	___ concern ______
n memory 'mem·o·ry	___ hiccups ______	___ suggestion ___
___ peppermint ______	___ newspaper ___	___ column ______
______	______	______

______________________ ________________ ________________

______________________ ________________ ________________

______________________ ________________ ________________

Now, let's focus on the meaning of these words. Read the list again. Put a check (✓) on the line to the left of all words you understand. Remember, finish this chapter and then return to this list. Check all new words you learned. In addition, write in other words you learned that are not on the list. Don't forget to review them often!

I. My Grandmother's Remedies

A. Read the passage.

When I was a young girl, my grandmother took care of me. She lived with my parents and me. When I was sick, she had many wonderful and strange remedies. These remedies helped me feel better. For a cold, she gave me peppermint candies and orange juice. For the hiccups, she fed me sugar on a spoon. My grandma was a wonderful person. She loved me very much.

My grandma is no longer alive, but I think about her every day. I often give my grandmother's remedies to other people: peppermint candies, orange juice, and love.

B. Answer the following questions about the passage.

1. Who did the grandmother live with?

2. What remedy did the grandma give for a cold?

3. Why did she feed sugar to the girl?

C. To form the simple past tense of a regular verb, you add *-ed* to the simple verb form. The same past tense form is used for all subjects (I, we, he, etc.).

Example:

ask The doctor *asked* a question.
They *asked* a question.

But to form the simple past tense of an irregular verb, you do not add *-ed* to the simple form of the verb. Spelling of irregular verbs is different. You must memorize these forms.

Example:

take My grandma *took* care of me.

The Simple Past Tense: Regular Verbs

Simple Verb Form	*Simple Past*
help	The remedies *helped* her.
listen	We *listened* to her advice.
answer	I *answered* the phone.

The Simple Past Tense: Irregular Verbs

Simple Verb Form	*Simple Past*
feed	My grandma *fed* me sugar.
sing	She *sang* songs every night.
drink	We *drank* ice tea in the sun.

D. In Activity A, underline all past tense verbs in the passage. Decide if each verb is regular or irregular and write the verb in the correct column. Then, write the correct base form of each verb. For words you do not know, use your dictionary. An example is provided. You will add more verbs to this list later.

Simple Past Tense: Regular	Base Form	Simple Past Tense: Irregular	Base Form
		was	be

E. Read the following paragraph and write the simple past tense form of each verb. If necessary, use your dictionary. Add any new words to the list you started in Activity D.

A Terrible Day

Yesterday (be) __was__ a terrible day. I (wake) __________ up 30 minutes late, and I (have) __________ a sore throat. To soothe my throat, I (make) __________ hot lemon tea. I quickly (drink) __________ the tea, and it (burn) __________ my tongue. Then, I (eat) __________ a quick breakfast and (leave) __________ for work. I (miss) __________ the bus, so I (start) __________ to walk. Soon, it (begin) __________ to rain! I (return) __________ home and (go) __________ back to bed. Hopefully, tomorrow will be a better day!

F. What did you do yesterday? Use the words to write complete sentences using the simple past tense.

Example:

make, appointment — I made a doctor's appointment.

1. go, dentist ______
2. complete, forms ______
3. take, medicine ______
4. call, doctor ______
5. eat, cafeteria ______
6. return, books ______
7. feed, baby ______

G. With another student, discuss ways to study and learn new irregular verbs. List three ways.

1.

2.

3.

II. International Remedies

A. Every country has its own unique home remedies. These remedies are passed down from generation to generation. In small groups, discuss home remedies from your country. First, describe and write the symptoms of each illness (what it feels like). Then, make a list of remedies or advice. Write in the countries for each remedy.

	Illness and Symptoms	Home Remedy and Country
1.	a sore throat My throat hurts. It hurts to swallow.	Drink lemon tea—Korea Eat honey—Saudi Arabia
2.	a headache	
3.	a cough	
4.	the hiccups	
5.	a cold	
6.	the flu	
7.	diarrhea	
8.	constipation	
9.	a stomachache	
10.	a toothache	

III. Dear Doctor

Many newspapers contain advice columns. When readers have social or health problems, they can write a letter to the newspaper column. The author of the column (the columnist) answers these letters. Some of these problems and their responses are printed in the newspaper. Then, people with the same problem can find help. These columns are often interesting and fun to read!

A. Quickly read the following letters and their responses.

Dear Doctor:
Last week, I got a cold. I went to buy some medicine, but I couldn't read the labels. I have studied English for only three months.Can you help me?
Yours very truly,
Can't Read Labels

Dear Can't Read Labels:
Do you have a cold? Maybe you don't need to take medicine, Instead, you can follow a simple home remedy. For example, you should drink orange juice every morning. You must get plenty of rest each night. You shouldn't stay up late. Follow this advice, and I hope you feel better.
Sincerely,
Doctor

Dear Doctor:
I moved to this country two months ago. For the past month, I have not felt well. I am always tired, but I sleep nine hours each night. I am very worried. What is wrong with me?
Yours very truly,
Concerned

Dear Concerned:
You may be depressed. Sleeping a lot is one symptom of depression. You must talk to a teacher, a classmate, or a counselor. Tell them your concerns. You should try to share your feelings. You can adjust to a new culture, but it takes time.
Sincerely,
Doctor

B. With advice, the modals *must* and *should* are often used. Return to the letters in Activity A. Quickly find and circle every *must* and *should*. In these letters, what is the difference between *must* and *should*?

<table>
<tr><td colspan="2">Modals of Advice: Must and Should</td></tr>
<tr><td colspan="2">The modals must and should are followed by the simple form of a verb.</td></tr>
<tr><td>For example:</td><td>She eats each day. → She must eat each day.
He calls his mother. → He should call his mother.
They go to the store. → They should go to the store.</td></tr>
<tr><td>Must</td><td>Something is a strong necessity. You don't have a choice.
Judy broke her leg. She must go to the hospital.
Nadia wants to see the movie. She must buy a ticket first.</td></tr>
<tr><td>Must not</td><td>Something is prohibited. It is important that you not do something. The negative form is must not. The contraction form is mustn't.
Khaled sprained his leg. He mustn't walk on it for two weeks.</td></tr>
<tr><td>Should</td><td>Something is suggested, but you make the choice.
Bill doesn't feel well. He should stay in bed.
You have a headache. You should take an aspirin.</td></tr>
<tr><td>Should not</td><td>Something is not suggested. It is advised that you not do something. The negative form is should not. The contraction form is shouldn't.
Maria has a sore throat. She shouldn't talk a lot.</td></tr>
</table>

C. Read these situations and complete each sentence with *must, should, mustn't,* or *shouldn't.* Sometimes more than one modal may be appropriate.

1. John is lonely. He ____________________ try to make new friends.
2. You ____________________ take medicine with alcohol.
3. So Jung broke her leg. She ____________________ see a doctor.
4. Irit went to the dentist. She ____________________ forget to pay her bill.

5. You ____________________ go to the doctor's office without an appointment.
6. Jorge failed his English classes. He ____________________ talk to his teacher.
7. Marika cut her hand. She ____________________ clean the wound.
8. Children ____________________ play with fire.
9. Emre is very tired. He ____________________ go to sleep.
10. Marty has a headache. He ____________________ listen to loud music.

D. Read the following letter. Then, pretend you are the doctor. Write a response for this column. Follow the letter format and punctuation used in Activity A.

Dear Doctor:

I miss my family and home country. When I arrived to America, I was excited and happy. Now, I am sad and depressed. Everything is different here. Students' customs are strange. My roommate is nice, but we are not good friends. Also, the food is not very good. I want to go home. What do you suggest?

Signed,
Having Problems

Dear Having Problems:

The Writing Process

Good writing is a long process. A good writer writes and rewrites a paragraph. A good writer asks others for suggestions. Many revisions (changes) are made in vocabulary, sentence use, and ideas.

E. Use the steps in the writing process to write a letter.

Step 1. Write a draft of a letter. Express a concern or problem. What is your problem or concern? How does it make you feel? Or write about an illness you had. What were the symptoms? What were your fears or concerns about the illness?

Step 2. When you finish your draft, show it to your teacher. Ask for comments about your writing (feedback). Is your letter easy to read? Are details used? Are the correct verb forms used?

Step 3. Use your teacher's suggestions and make appropriate revisions. Rewrite your letter.

Step 4. Finally, exchange your letter with a classmate. Your classmate will pretend to be a doctor. He or she will write a response to your letter.

Chapter 4

The Doctor's Office

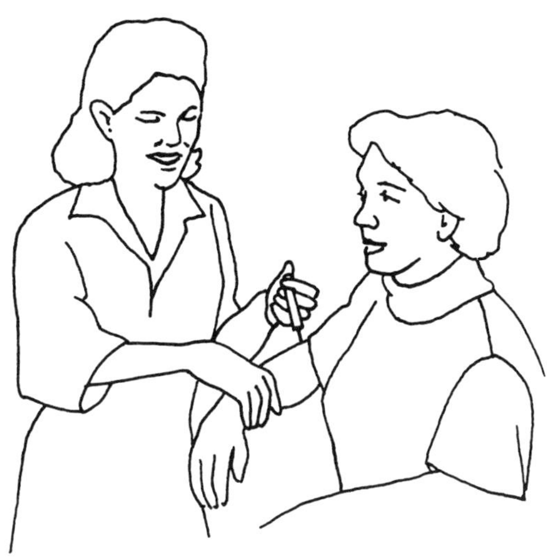

A Look Behind/A Look Ahead

In chapter 3, you learned about home remedies for common or minor illnesses. But sometimes an illness is not minor. It is serious. For a serious illness, a home remedy will not help you. Instead, you should see a doctor. Thousands of Americans visit a doctor each year. They see a doctor because they are sick. Or they see a doctor for a checkup (a general medical examination). At a checkup, the doctor checks for possible illnesses. The doctor also gives health advice or treatment.

This chapter provides the basic information and language skills needed to choose and visit a doctor.

To the Student

After completing this chapter, you will

1. understand what happens at a doctor's office in the United States,
2. be able to find a doctor for your needs, and
3. be able to make an appointment to see a doctor.

Vocabulary Development

In English, there are many common word beginnings (prefixes) and word endings (suffixes).

Example:

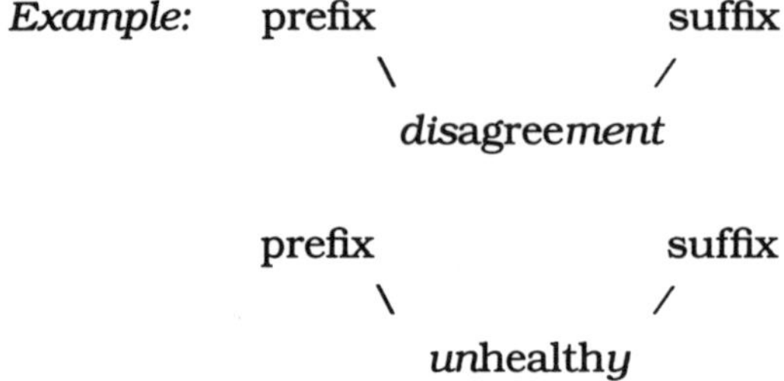

Prefixes and suffixes help define words.

Example:

Dis- and *un-* are prefixes for "not." The word *disagreement* means not in agreement; the word *unhealthy* means not healthy.

Prefixes and suffixes also show what part of speech a word is.

Example:

-ment is a noun suffix, so the word *disagreement* is a noun.
-y is an adjective suffix, so the word *unhealthy* is an adjective.

Many suffixes can be added to words to change their part of speech.

Example:

Add *-ment* to the verb *disagree* to form the noun *disagreement.*
Add *-y* to the noun *health* to form the adjective *healthy.*

The following suffixes are attached to nouns: *-ment, -er, -or, -ist, -ion,* and *-ian.* Scan the following list of words for these suffixes and circle them.

Then, use your dictionary to determine the part of speech for each word. Write the part of speech on the line. The first two are done for you.

__ appointment n	__ checkup ______	__ directory ______
__ forms n	__ history ______	__ physician ______
__ medicine ______	__ nurse ______	__ patient ______
__ pharmacy ______	__ prescription ______	__ receptionist ______
__ specialist ______	__ aspirin ______	__ sprain ______
______	______	______
______	______	______
______	______	______
______	______	______

Now, focus on word meaning. Put a check (✓) on the line to the left of all the words you understand. Finish this chapter and return to this list. Check all the new words you learned. In addition, add any other words you learned that are not on the list. Don't forget to review them often!

I. Call the Doctor

A. Before you read the passage in Activity C called "Oh, My Aching Back," think about your answers to these questions.

1. When should you go to a doctor?
2. Why should you make an appointment before you see a doctor?
3. What questions might a doctor or other medical people ask you?
4. How do you find an appropriate doctor for your needs?

B. Scan the passage in Activity C to put the events in the correct order. Read to find the information needed. Do not read all of the passage. The first one is done for you.

According to the story, Michael ________________________.

_______ went to the pharmacy

_______ made a doctor's appointment

___1___ helped a friend move

_______ took some medication

_______ felt better

_______ went to the doctor's office

_______ completed medical forms

C. Now, read the passage carefully.

Oh, My Aching Back!

Last weekend, Michael helped his friend move into a new apartment. For two hours, they carried many heavy boxes and some furniture. "That was hard work, but it's nice to help a friend," thought Michael.

The next morning, however, Michael woke with a sore back. He thought the pain would go away with aspirin and a warm shower, but it didn't. A week later, his back still hurt. "I must see a doctor," Michael told his wife. That morning, he called the health center. The receptionist answered the phone.

"I'd like to make an appointment to see a doctor," stated Michael.

The receptionist asked what was wrong. After the receptionist got this information, she said, "We'll see you on Thursday at 10:00 A.M. Please arrive 15 minutes early. All new patients must complete medical forms."

On Thursday, Michael arrived at the doctor's office. He talked with the receptionist. He also completed some forms. The forms asked about his medical history and health insurance.

Fifteen minutes later, a nurse called his name, "Michael Ravis? Please follow me." The nurse led Michael to a small examination room. She asked him some questions about his pain. She also took his temperature and checked his blood pressure. "The doctor will be with you in a few moments," she said.

Soon the doctor entered the room. Michael explained his problem to Dr. Fowler while she examined him.

"You've strained your back, Michael," Dr. Fowler announced.

"Sprained?" Michael questioned.

"No, strained. It isn't as serious as a sprain, but the pain can still be very strong. I will prescribe a muscle relaxer and mild painkiller. You should also take it easy for a while. You can buy the prescription at the pharmacy downstairs. If you still have pain in two weeks, you should make another appointment to see me."

Michael took the prescription to the pharmacy. He bought the medicine. He followed the doctor's orders and soon felt much better. "A visit to the doctor was easier than I thought," Michael told his wife. "I'm glad I went!"

D. Sometimes, you can guess the meaning of many words from context. For example, study the sentence, "The *receptionist* answered the phone." You can guess that a receptionist is a person who answers phones. In the passage, locate each of the following words. Reread the sentences. Then, match each word with the best definition.

1. ______ appointment		a. a drug used to treat an illness or pain
2. ______ forms		b. a store where medicine is prepared and sold
3. ______ history		c. a meeting at a certain time and place
4. __h__ receptionist		d. events of the past
5. ______ medicine		e. papers with blanks for answers and information

6. ______ nurse — f. a person who receives medical care

7. ______ patient — g. a person who is trained to care for sick people

8. ______ pharmacy — h. a person who greets people and answers phones for a business

9. ______ prescription — i. a doctor's written order for medicine

E. Decide whether these sentences are true (T) or false (F). Then, rewrite the false sentences to make them true.

Example:

__F__ Michael helped his friend move, and he hurt his ~~leg.~~ back

______ 1. Michael completed forms at the doctor's office.

______ 2. The receptionist brought Michael to an examination room.

______ 3. The nurse took the patient's temperature and checked his blood pressure.

______ 4. Michael sprained his back.

______ 5. The doctor gave Michael some medicine.

F. Select the *best* answer to the following questions. Try to answer without looking at the passage.

1. What remedies did Michael use before he went to the doctor?
   a. nothing—he thought the pain would go away
   b. aspirin and a warm shower
   c. medicine from the pharmacy

2. What does a receptionist do?
   a. schedules appointments and greets patients
   b. brings patients to the examination rooms
   c. prescribes medicine
3. Michael completed forms about his ____________________.
   a. temperature and blood pressure
   b. medical history and insurance
   c. medical and employment history
4. The doctor advised Michael to ____________________.
   a. take medicine and rest
   b. not lift heavy boxes and furniture
   c. see another doctor in two weeks

G. In chapter 3, you studied regular and irregular verb forms. Look at the passage in Activity C and circle all simple past tense verbs. Which verbs are regular? Which verbs are irregular? Write each verb in the correct column. Then, write the base form. For words you do not know, use your dictionary. (The chart continues on page 52.)

Simple Past Tense: Regular	Base Form	Simple Past Tense: Irregular	Base Form

Simple Past Tense: Regular	Base Form	Simple Past Tense: Irregular	Base Form

H. On a sheet of paper, combine this list and your list from chapter 3 (p. 38). Put all verbs in alphabetical order. Review them often.

I. Write a paragraph describing an illness you had. Explain what you did. Did you go to the doctor? Did you use a home remedy? When you are finished, check the paragraph for sentence structure and the use of past tense verbs.

II. Choosing a Doctor

It can be confusing to find an appropriate doctor. But it does not have to be. Most doctors are listed in the telephone book. In addition, insurance companies provide a directory of doctors. This directory lists doctors in your area. Finally, your school or office may have a health center. A health center provides basic medical care for students and/or workers and their spouses. In the United States, people will see a general practitioner for a checkup. However, most doctors are specialists. Specialists have special knowledge in an area of medicine.

A. Read the list of specialists. Match the doctor on the left with the description on the right. Do not use a dictionary. Instead, look at the prefixes and suffixes for clues. They can help you understand the definitions.

Word Parts: Prefixes and Suffixes

pharm-	=	drug	psych-	=	mind
gyn-	=	female	opto-	=	vision (see)
dent-	=	tooth	-ist, -ian, -eon, -er	=	person
derm-	=	skin	-try, -ology	=	study of
pod-	=	foot			

		Specialist Titles		*Descriptions*
______	1.	optometrist	a.	professional who prepares and sells medicine
______	2.	pharmacist	b.	doctor who performs operations (surgery)
______	3.	pediatrician	c.	doctor for pregnant women
______	4.	surgeon	d.	foot doctor
______	5.	gynecologist	e.	teeth doctor
______	6.	obstetrician	f.	doctor for mental/ emotional concerns
______	7.	dentist	g.	skin doctor
______	8.	dermatologist	h.	women's doctor
______	9.	plastic surgeon	i.	eye doctor
______	10.	psychiatrist	j.	doctor who changes people's face and body
d	11.	podiatrist	k.	children's doctor

B. In the first column, write the title of the specialist needed for the situation given. Then, scan the medical directory. In the second column, write the first and the last name of the appropriate doctor. Work as fast as you can.

Specialist Title	*Doctor's First and Last Name*

Example:

You have a question about some medicine.

pharmacist	Erin Emre

MEDICAL DIRECTORY

Alper, Zachary DO
1540 Montreal Road
Decatur, GA . . . 354-5900
Plastic Surgeon

Brady, Donna OD
1402 Ponce de Leon Ave
Clarkston, GA . . . 567-2720
Optometry

Douglas, Amber DO PC
1601 W Peachtree
Atlanta, GA . . . 566-1406
Dermatology

Emre, Erin
1929 Memorial Drive
Atlanta, GA . . . 364-0404
Pharmacist

Frederick, Alvin MD
125 Sunset Drive
Lithonia, GA . . . 354-8672
Psychiatry

Klingaman, Sharla MD
4218 Bordeaux
Chamblee, GA . . . 566-5242
Obstetrician

Larson, Judith MD
1581 Forest Hills Road
Decatur, GA . . . 354-5460
Pediatrician

Luedtke, Paul DO
139 Coleridge Drive
Decatur, GA . . . 343-2912
Surgeon

Nelson, Walter DPM
871 Pine Street
Doraville, GA . . . 343-7527
Podiatrist

Robert, Marshall
4162 Candler Road
Lithonia, GA . . . 364-1976
Dentistry

Waddell, Joan MD
313 Frederick Avenue
Chamblee, GA . . . 566-8182
General Practitioner

Wald, Cathy MD
1922 Atherton Way
Buckhead, GA . . . 567-3112
Gynecology

1. Your spouse needs eyeglasses.

_______________ _______________

2. You have a bad toothache.

_______________ _______________

3. Your mother needs an operation.

_______________ _______________

4. Your young child is very sick.

______________________ ______________________

5. Your sister is having female problems.

______________________ ______________________

6. Your brother has a skin rash.

______________________ ______________________

7. You are sad all the time.

______________________ ______________________

8. You want to change the shape of your nose.

______________________ ______________________

9. Your sister-in-law is going to have a baby.

______________________ ______________________

10. Your father is having problems with his feet.

______________________ ______________________

III. Making an Appointment

A. After you select a doctor, you will need to make an appointment. Return to section I, "Call the Doctor," and read about Michael Ravis again. In the passage "Oh, My Aching Back!" Michael made an appointment to see Dr. Fowler. Now, listen to a new conversation with Michael and the receptionist at his doctor's office. You may not understand every word. Just listen for the main ideas. You may take notes on a sheet of paper.

B. Read the following words. Discuss the meaning of each word with a classmate.

daytime	forms	helped
opening	patient	regular
before	first	spell
history	victory	card
appointment		

C. Now, listen to the conversation again. Write the missing words in the correct blanks.

Receptionist: Dr. Fowler's office. How can I help you?

Michael: This is Michael Ravis. I'd like to make an ________________ to see the doctor.

Receptionist: All right. Are you a new ________________?

Michael: Ah, what do you mean?

Receptionist: Have you seen Dr. Fowler ________________?

Michael: Oh. No, I haven't.

Receptionist: Okay. Why do you need an appointment?

Michael: I ________________ a friend move a week ago, and now I have a sore back. Also, I should have a ________________ checkup. I haven't seen a doctor for two years.

Receptionist: Let's see. We have an ________________ for Thursday at 2:50 P.M.

Michael: 2:15?

Receptionist: No, 2:50. Ah, 10 minutes to 3.

Michael: Oh, that's fine.

Receptionist: Now, let me get some information. Can you ________________ your name for me, please?

Michael:	Sure, my ____________ name is Michael. My last name's Ravis. That's R, A, V, I, S.
Receptionist:	R, A, B, I, F?
Michael:	No, R, A, V as in ____________, I, S as in *smile.*
Receptionist:	Okay, and your ____________ phone number, please.
Michael:	752-7053.
Receptionist:	All right, we'll see you on Thursday at 2:50. Oh, Michael, please arrive 15 minutes early. There are some ____________ you'll need to complete.
Michael:	Some what?
Receptionist:	Some forms about your medical ____________.
Michael:	Oh, okay. Thank you. I'll see you on Thursday.
Receptionist:	Have a good day.

Intonation

When we speak, our voices rise and fall. This is called intonation. Intonation expresses feelings or questions. There are different situations for intonation.

Raise your voice to confirm that you heard the correct information.

My appointment is at 8:15?

Raise your voice when you ask a yes/no question.

Do you want to make an appointment?

However, make your voice fall when you ask an information question.

What is wrong with you?

D. Listen to the dialogue of Michael and the receptionist again. Draw an arrow to show where Michael's or the receptionist's voice rises or falls.

Michael:	This is Michael Ravis. I'd like to make an appointment to see a doctor.
Receptionist:	Which doctor would you like to see?
Michael:	Dr. Fowler, if she is available.
Receptionist:	Okay, let's see. We have an appointment for Thursday at 2:50 P.M.
Michael:	2:15?
Receptionist:	No, 2:50. Ah, 10 minutes to 3.

Listen to another dialogue of Michael and the receptionist. Draw an arrow to show where the receptionist's voice rises or falls.

Receptionist:	Can you spell your name for me, please?
Michael:	Sure, my first name is Michael. My last name's Ravis. That's R, A, V, I, S.
Receptionist:	R, A, B, I, F?
Michael:	No, R, A, V as in *victory*, I, S as in *smile.*

E. Following is a dialogue between a patient and a receptionist. Read and complete the dialogue. Draw an arrow to show where rising or falling intonation is necessary.

Receptionist:	This is Dr. Hill's office. May I help you?
Patient:	Yes, my name is ____________________, and I'd like to make an appointment with Dr. Hill.
Receptionist:	Are you a new patient?
Patient:	No, I'm not.
Receptionist:	Let me check our files. Okay, why do you want to see the doctor?
Patient:	I get headaches when I read. I might need stronger glasses.

Receptionist: Okay, how's ____________________ at ____________________?

Patient: I have class then. Do you have an earlier opening?

Receptionist: Ah, yes, we do. How's ____________________?

Patient: That's perfect.

Receptionist: Okay, what is your daytime phone number?

Patient: It's 651-2942.

Receptionist: Great! We'll see you on ____________________ at ____________________.

Patient: Thank you!

F. To make an appointment, you need to provide information (name, phone number, address). You need to ask and answer questions. Work with a partner. Together, write and practice a dialogue. Change intonation where necessary.

Student A:
You recently moved to this country and don't feel well. Call a doctor to make an appointment for the first time. Describe your symptoms to the receptionist.

It is often difficult to understand pronunciation over the telephone. You may need to spell or repeat words. A useful tip is to follow this pattern: "My name is SuFen. That's S, U, F as in *friend*, E, N as in *no*." (The word *friend* begins with the letter *F* and the word *no* begins with the letter *N*.)

Student B:
You are the receptionist for Dr. Barry's office. Record the information on the following chart. You might need to ask the patient to spell or repeat words. You can ask: "How do you spell that?" or "Can you repeat that?" The information you receive helps the doctor. With this information, the doctor can provide the best care for the patient. *You should always print the information on a form.*

1. Name ______________________________

   Address ______________________________

   ____

   Daytime phone number ______________________________

2. Date of birth ______________________________

3. Illness and symptoms

4. Medical history

5. Appointment date and time ______________________________

When you finish, switch roles. Practice being both the patient and the receptionist.

The next time you visit a doctor, bring this information with you. It will help you complete your doctor's forms. It also may make your visit easier and less stressful.

Chapter 5

Medications

Draw a line to connect each label direction to the appropriate medication.

Take 2 *capsules* every 8 hours as needed.
Take one spoonful of *syrup* with each meal.
Rub *cream* on rash each day.
Take 1 *tablet* daily.
Use 2 *lozenges* when throat is sore. Dissolve in mouth.

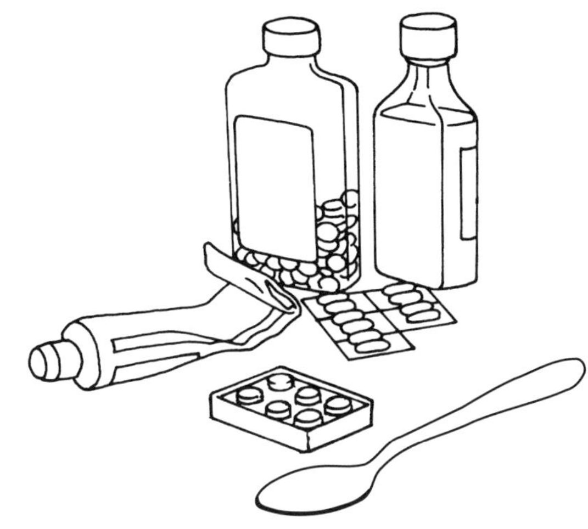

A Look Behind/A Look Ahead

In chapter 4, you learned how to communicate with your doctor or other medical people. When you are sick, your doctor may want you to take medication. There are many different types of medications. They include capsules, tablets, syrups, lozenges, and creams. It is important for you to read and understand the labels of these medicines.

Chapter 5 provides the information and language skills needed to understand and follow medicine labels. This chapter also teaches you how to carefully buy medicine.

To the Student

After completing this chapter, you will

1. understand the difference between prescription and over-the-counter drug products,
2. understand the labels of drug products, and
3. know how to protect yourself against drug products that have been tampered with.

Vocabulary Development

Put a check (✓) on the line to the left of all the words you understand. Write the part of speech for each word to the right. The first two words are done for you. When you finish this chapter, return to this list. Check additional words you learned. Then, add any new words you learned that are not on the list. Review them often!

___ over-the-counter drug __n__	___ discard ______	___ dosage ______
___ relieve __v__	___ expiration date ____	___ tamper ______
___ label ______	___ prescription drug __	___ refill ______
___ side effect ______	___ warning ______	___ FDA ______
___ tablet ______	___ capsule ______	___ syrup ______
______	______	______
______	______	______
______	______	______
______	______	______

I. The Pharmacy

A. Think about your answers to these questions.

1. If a doctor advises you to take medication, what questions should you ask?
2. In the United States, where do you buy medication?
3. What information is provided on medication labels?
4. Are all legal drugs safe to take?
5. What laws does your native country have for legal drug products?

B. Amy Lee is not feeling well. She visits her doctor's office and then the local pharmacy. Listen to Amy's conversation in the dictation. Then, answer the questions.

1. What is wrong with Amy?

2. What did the doctor do for Amy?

3. What did Amy ask the pharmacist?

C. Listen to the next part of the dictation. The pharmacist explains the parts of a prescription drug label. Find these parts on the label. Write the parts on the lines provided.

prescription number	expiration date of medicine
medication directions	pharmacy information
patient's name	name and amount of medicine in package

1. ______________________ CARES PHARMACY 212 PEACH ST. ATLANTA, GA PHONE: 404-882-1930
2. ______________________ Rx# 10015288 FOSTER, J.
3. ______________________ AMY LEE
4. ______________________ TAKE 1 TABLET TWICE A DAY.
5. ______________________ EXP 3-98
6. ______________________ 60 FIBROZILT TAB 600 MG

4 REFILLS

D. Use the information from the conversation and the label to select the *best* answer to the following questions.

1. What is the phone number of the pharmacy?

   a. 326-8100

   b. 882-1930

2. The prescription number is needed for a refill. A refill means ____________________.

   a. different medicine

   b. more medicine

3. How much medication should Amy take each day?

   a. 2 tablets

   b. 1 tablet

4. How much medicine is in this prescription bottle?

   a. 60 tablets

   b. 600 tablets

5. Discard the medicine after the expiration date. Discard means ____________________.

   a. get new medicine

   b. throw away the medicine

E. Listen carefully to the next part of the dictation. The pharmacist explains the difference between prescription and over-the-counter drug products. Respond to the following statements with true (T) or false (F). Then, correct the false statements so that they are true.

Example:

__F__ Over-the-counter drugs ~~are not~~ *can be* very effective.

Over-the-counter drug products

______ 1. are bought from your doctor.

_______ 2. can relieve the symptoms of all illnesses.

_______ 3. can be bought without a prescription.

II. Over-the-Counter Medications

A. Nine out of ten Americans take care of their everyday aches and pains. They do not see a health professional with these problems. They do nothing, use a home remedy, or buy an over-the-counter (OTC) drug product. They like to take care of themselves. Can you think of any OTC products? List them in the space provided.

B. Read the passage.

Safe and Sure Self-Care with Over-the-Counter Medicines

Over-the-counter drug products must be used properly. You must read the label carefully. You must follow the instructions carefully. In the United States, there is a government organization. This organization makes medications safe. The organization is called the Food and Drug Administration (FDA). The FDA says OTC labels must give certain information.

The following information should appear on any OTC drug label.

The product name and the drug type. Examples of drug types include tablets, capsules, and cream.

Warnings. Warnings tell people with medical problems (like high blood pressure or heart disease) not to take the medicine. They also tell possible side effects such as excitability or drowsiness (sleepiness). Other warnings include: "Keep all drugs away from children" and "If you are pregnant, don't use this product."

Instructions for use. This explains how much medicine to take (dosage), when to take it, and how to take it. ("Tablet should be chewed." "Take with water or food.")

Tamper-safe containers. This makes the product safer. The package shows when someone tampers with the medicine. It might say: "Tamper-safe bottle cap. If seal is broken, do not use." You should check all packages. Packages should not be open, cut, or broken.

The expiration date. After this month and year, the drug might not work as well. An outdated (old) drug may not provide relief. In fact, it could be harmful. Discard the medicine after this date.

Source: Adapted from *Safe and Sure Self-Care with Over-the-Counter Medicines*, Department of Health and Human Services, Food and Drug Administration, DHHS Publication No. (FDA) 92–3198, 1992.

C. Match the following words with their definitions. Use the information from the previous listening and reading activities.

______	1.	prescription drugs	a.	the month and year that the drug should no longer be taken
______	2.	a label	b.	medicine you buy without a doctor's permission
______	3.	to tamper	c.	information about the product
______	4.	to discard	d.	more medicine
______	5.	a dosage	e.	medicine a doctor must prescribe
______	6.	a warning	f.	to change without permission
______	7.	the expiration date	g.	information of something bad that may happen
______	8.	side effects	h.	to reduce pain or worries
______	9.	to relieve	i.	the amount of medicine to take
______	10.	a refill	j.	to throw away
______	11.	over-the-counter drugs	k.	things that can happen after taking, e.g., drowsiness

D. Use words from Activity C and fill in the blanks in these sentences.

1. Do not drink this milk; the ______________________ was last week.
2. You do not need a doctor's prescription to buy ______________ ______________.
3. When we are thirsty, we go to the restaurant on the corner. Buy one cola, and all ______________________ are free!
4. Read the ______________________ to learn what is in this can of soup.
5. Do not ______________________ with medication and food products. It is against the law.

E. Complete these sentences in your own words.

1. Two *side effects* of drinking alcohol are ______________ ______________.
2. I was very *relieved* when ______________________.
3. My father *warned* me about ______________________.
4. Every spring we clean our apartment. We *discard* ______________ ______________________________.
5. ______________________ can tell you the proper *dosage* of your medicine.

F. Return to the passage in Activity B and read it again. Then, decide whether these sentences are true (T) or false (F). Finally, in the passage, underline or highlight the sentences that contain the correct answers.

_______ 1. The FDA makes medications safe.

_______ 2. Medicine cannot get old.

_______ 3. Sleepiness is a possible side effect of some medications.

_______ 4. Some labels tell people to take the medication with food or drink.

_______ 5. Tamper-safe containers protect medicine.

G. Use the information from the passage in Activity B and identify the following information on this over-the-counter drug label.

name of product
type of drug
tamper-safe container
warnings
instructions for use
expiration date

EXTRA STRENGTH
TYLENOL®
Strong Pain Relief
Contains No Aspirin
Gelcaps
acetaminophen
50 SOLID GELCAPS – 500 MG EACH
Gelatin Coated
EXTRA STRENGTH
TYLENOL®
Gelcaps
acetaminophen
McNEIL
McNEIL CONSUMER PRODUCTS CO.
DIVISION OF McNEIL-PPC, INC.
FORT WASHINGTON, PA 19034 USA

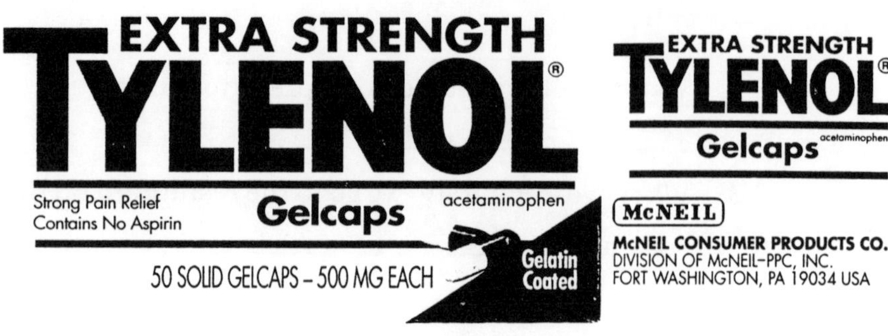

USUAL DOSAGE: Adults and Children 12 years of Age and Older: Two gelcaps 3 or 4 times daily. No more than a total of 8 gelcaps in any 24-hour period.

INACTIVE INGREDIENTS: Benzyl Alcohol, Butylparaben, Castor Oil, Cellulose, Corn Starch, Edetate Calcium Disodium, Gelatin, Hydroxypropyl Methylcellulose, Magnesium Stearate, Methylparaben, Propylparaben, Sodium Lauryl Sulfate, Sodium Propionate, Sodium Starch Glycolate, Titanium Dioxide, Blue #1 and #2, Red #40 and Yellow #10.

WARNING: DO NOT USE IF CARTON IS OPENED OR PRINTED RED NECK WRAP OR PRINTED FOIL INNER SEAL IS BROKEN. DO NOT TAKE FOR PAIN FOR MORE THAN 10 DAYS OR FOR FEVER FOR MORE THAN 3 DAYS UNLESS DIRECTED BY A PHYSICIAN. SEVERE OR RECURRENT PAIN OR HIGH OR CONTINUED FEVER MAY BE INDICATIVE OF SERIOUS ILLNESS. UNDER THESE CONDITIONS, CONSULT A PHYSICIAN. KEEP THIS AND ALL MEDICATION OUT OF THE REACH OF CHILDREN. AS WITH ANY DRUG, IF YOU ARE PREGNANT OR NURSING A BABY, SEEK THE ADVICE OF A HEALTH PROFESSIONAL BEFORE USING THIS PRODUCT. IN THE CASE OF ACCIDENTAL OVERDOSAGE, CONTACT A PHYSICIAN OR POISON CONTROL CENTER IMMEDIATELY.

See end panel for expiration date. Store at room temperature; avoid high humidity and excessive heat 40°C (104°F).

Patent 4,820,524. ©McN-PPC, Inc. '93

3 0045-0468-50 5
EXP: 08/95

III. Medicine Labels

At the supermarket, you see many types of medications. You see many different boxes and bottles in various sizes and colors. When you buy medication, you don't want to read every label. That would take too much time. Instead, you should scan for the information you need.

A. Read the following questions about drug labels and scan for the appropriate information. Find the information quickly.

Label 1

ALP PHARMACIES
125 SUNSET BLVD.
MADISON, WI
PHONE: 608-752-7058

Rx# 868261001 LARSON, J.
SHARLA KLINGAMAN
TAKE 2 TABLETS DAILY.

EXP 5-98

45 VAZOTELK TAB 500MG
3 REFILLS

1. What is the name of this medication?

2. Is this an over-the-counter drug or a prescription drug?

3. Where can a person buy this medicine?

4. What kind of a drug is this? (e.g., tablet, capsule, syrup, ointment)

5. How much medication should an adult take at one time?

6. How often should a patient take this medication?

7. When should a person discard this medication?

8. How much medicine is in this package?

Label 2

12 HOUR
COLDTAB

10 CAPSULES

- Sneezing
- Runny Nose
- Itchy Eyes
- Nasal Congestion

UP TO 12 HOURS OF TEMPORARY RELIEF, WITHOUT DROWSINESS

Indications: For the temporary relief of nasal congestion due to the common cold, allergies, or hay fever, including runny nose, sneezing, and itchy eyes.
Directions: Adults and children 12 years and older: Take one capsule every 12 hours, not to exceed 2 capsules in 24 hours. Children under 12 years old: Consult a doctor.
Warnings: May cause nervousness, dizziness, or sleeplessness. Do not take with alcoholic beverages. Do not take this product if you have high blood pressure or diabetes. Do not take this product for more than 7 days.

Keep this and all drugs out of the reach of children.

This is not a real product.

1. What is the name of this drug?

2. Can you buy this medicine without a prescription?

3. What does this medicine soothe?

4. What kind of a drug is this? (e.g., syrup, ointment)

5. How much medication should a 13-year-old child take each day?

6. How often should a child over 12 years take this medication?

7. List two warnings of this medicine.

8. How much medicine is in this box?

B. Read these sentences from medication labels.

Take as directed.
Keep all medicine out of reach of children.
Repeat every hour as needed.

These sentences illustrate the use of the imperative. Each sentence begins with the simple verb form: take, keep, repeat. No subject is provided. In each of these sentences, what is the subject? In other words, who should take all medications as directed, keep all medicine away from children, and repeat the process every hour? (Read "The Imperative" if you need help.)

The subject is ______________________________

The Imperative

- When you use the imperative, the subject *you* (singular or plural) is not given; it is understood.
- Use an imperative verb (simple form) to give instructions or directions, to give a command, or to make a request (usually with *please*).
- When you use the negative imperative, use *do not* or *don't* before the verb.

C. Find four examples of imperative verbs on the labels in Activity A. Write the sentences here:

1. ______________________________
2. ______________________________
3. ______________________________
4. ______________________________

D. Study the following examples of imperative sentences. Where might you hear or read these sentences? Write your answers on the lines.

Example:

Please do not talk during the movie.
Pick up trash before leaving. ______Signs at a movie theater.______

1. Write your name on the paper.
   Read each item carefully.
   Please don't talk during the test. ______________________________
2. Check to see if person is breathing.
   Dial 911 for emergency help. ______________________________

3. Turn left at the corner.
   Go three blocks to the stop light. ____________________
4. Drive carefully.
   Do not enter. ____________________
5. Don't use alcohol with this medication.
   Take with juice or water. ____________________

E. Write the steps to take when you feel ill. Use the imperative verb form. Two possible steps are provided for you.

   1. Call your doctor's office.
   2. Explain your illness to the receptionist.
   3. ____________________
   4. ____________________
   5. ____________________

F. On a piece of paper, write the instructions or directions for one of the following. Use the imperative verb form.

   How to get to your home from school or work
   How to improve your English vocabulary
   How to care for a cut on your finger
   How to . . .

IV. Tamper-Safe Products

A. How can you protect yourself against tampered drug products? Stop, look, and look again! Read the pamphlet, *Buying Medicine? Stop, Look, Look Again.* This pamphlet was written by the U.S. FDA and the Non-Prescription Drug Manufacturers Association. When you have finished reading the pamphlet, go back and circle all the imperative verbs.

Buying Medicine? Stop, Look, Look Again

HELP PROTECT YOURSELF AGAINST TAMPERING

Before you buy it take a look; before you take it look again.

U.S. nonprescription, over-the-counter (OTC) medicines are among the most safely packaged consumer products in the world. Most **by law** are sealed in **tamper-evident** packaging for your protection. But manufacturers cannot make a tamper-**proof** package. They can only make the safest package that technology allows. The rest is up to you.

You can help protect yourself

Here's how:

- **Read the label.** OTC medicines with tamper-evident packages tell you on the label what seals and other features you should look for.
- Inspect the outer packaging. **Look before you buy it!**
- Inspect the medicine itself when you open the package. Look again before you take it! **If it looks suspicious, be suspicious.**
- Look especially for capsules or tablets that are **different in any way** from others in the package.
- Don't use any medicine from a package that shows cuts, slices, tears or other imperfections.
- Never take medicines in the dark.
- Read the label and look at the medicine **every time** you take a dose.

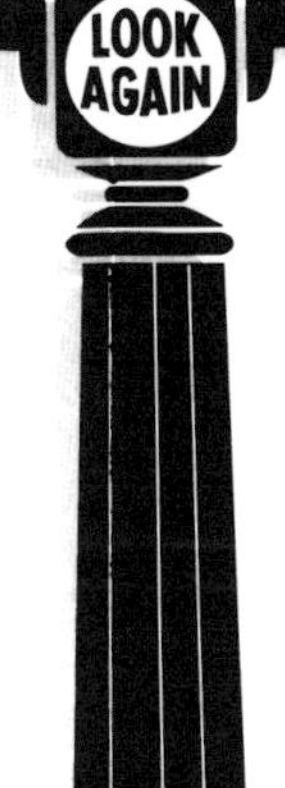

If in doubt tell somebody

Not every change in the appearance or condition of a product means that it has been tampered with. But if there is any question in your mind, don't buy it, don't use it and don't leave it at that. **Tell somebody** who can do something about it!

Whenever you suspect anything wrong with a medicine or its packaging, take it back to the store. If there is a real problem, the manager will report it to the proper authorities.

Remember

No one can **prevent** tampering. What tamper-evident packaging does is try to provide evidence of tampering that you can see **if you look.**

What you can do is pay attention to the safety features that the manufacturer has provided. With a little time, a little care and your own good sense you can be the best safety feature of all.

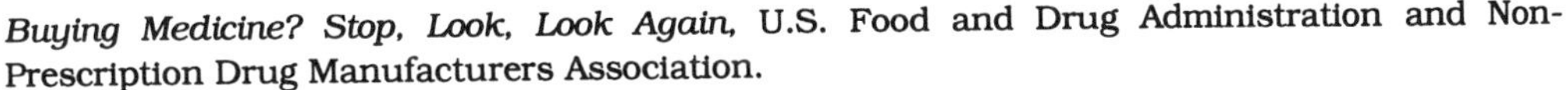

Buying Medicine? Stop, Look, Look Again, U.S. Food and Drug Administration and Non-Prescription Drug Manufacturers Association.

B. Circle the letter that best describes the main idea of the pamphlet. The main idea is the general idea of the pamphlet.

a. You should read labels carefully.

b. You should buy and use medicine carefully.

The correct answer is b. You must do more than read a label carefully. To protect yourself against tampered drugs, you must do many things. Reading the label is one of those things.

C. In the pamphlet, some ideas explain or support the main idea (buy and use medicine carefully). For example, "Read the label" supports the main idea. This is one supporting detail. Find additional supporting details and underline them.

Main Idea and Supporting Details

- The main idea is the general idea of the text.
- The supporting details explain or support the main idea.
- Large print, **bold print,** or <u>underlined print</u> helps you understand important ideas.

D. Look back at the pamphlet on page 73. Count the imperative verb forms you circled. How many did you find? ____________________

Chapter 6

Basic Nutrition

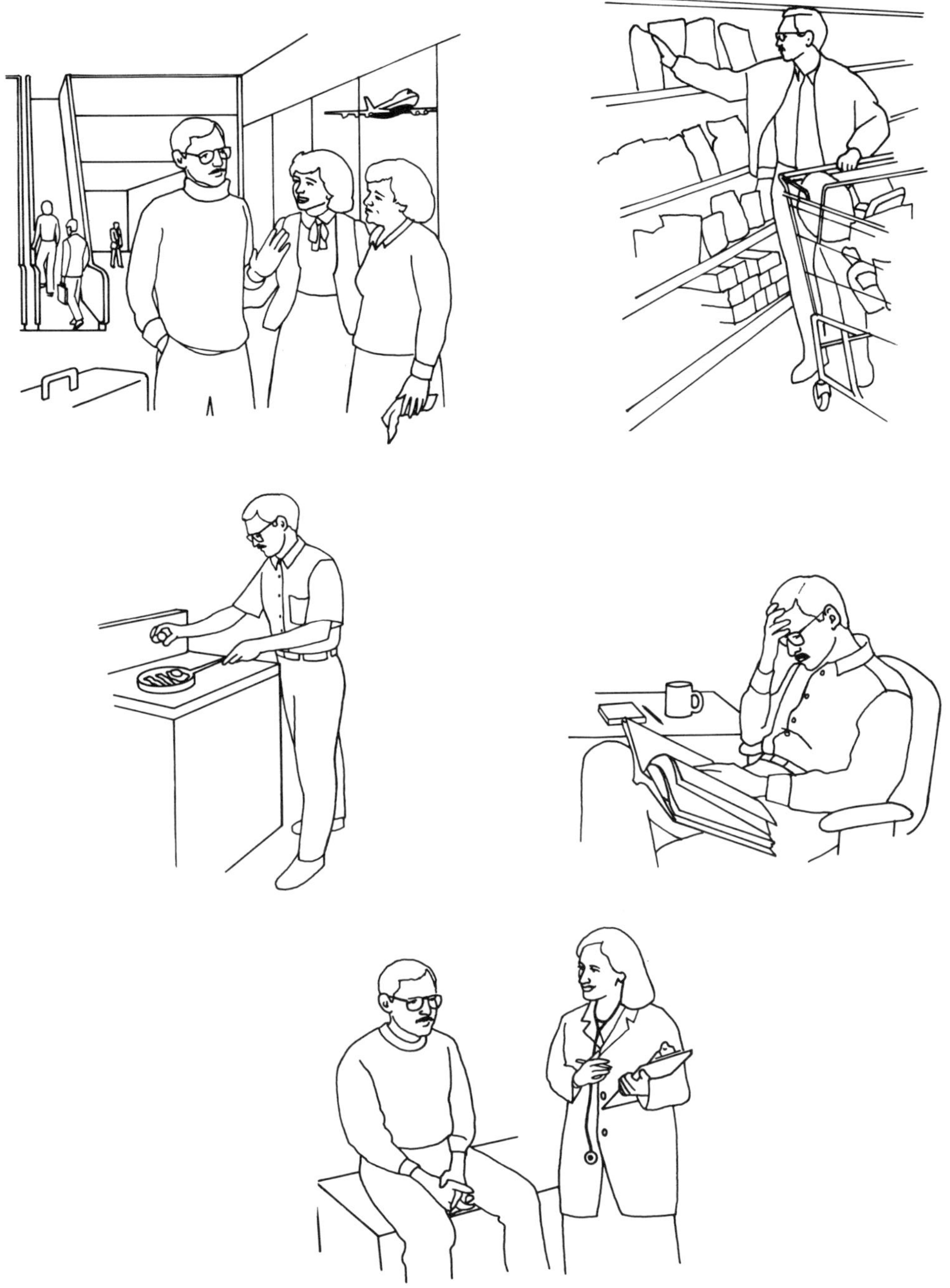

A Look Behind/A Look Ahead

In chapter 5, you learned to read and understand medicine labels. You also learned to be careful when you buy new products. This is important when you buy medicine products. But it is also important when you buy food products.

In American supermarkets, there are many different food products. It is difficult to choose the best items. Food labels may be unfamiliar. Sometimes, labels are difficult to understand.

Chapter 6 explains food labels. It also helps you understand healthy eating habits.

To the Student

After completing this chapter, you will

1. understand the Food Guide Pyramid,
2. understand the Nutrition Facts on food labels, and
3. understand how to make smart food choices in supermarkets, fast food restaurants, and cafeterias.

Vocabulary Development

Put a check (✓) on the line to the left of all the words you understand. Write the part of speech to the right. The first two have been done for you. When you finish this chapter, return to this list. Write in additional words you learned. Don't forget to review this list.

__ serving __n__	__ habits ______	__ supermarket ______
__ ingredient __n__	__ cafeteria ______	__ fast food ______
__ brand name ______	__ pyramid ______	__ nutrient ______
__ calorie ______	__ food log ______	__ nutrition ______
__ energy ______	__ habit ______	__ bread ______
__ bag ______	__ fat ______	__ sugar ______
__ fruit ______	__ slice ______	__ milk ______

___ meat ____________	___ vegetable ____________	___ package ____________
____________	____________	____________
____________	____________	____________
____________	____________	____________
____________	____________	____________

I. Healthy Eating Habits

A. Look at the pictures at the beginning of this chapter. With a classmate, decide what Roberto is doing in each picture. Underneath each picture, write a sentence to describe what is happening. Use the present progressive verb form.

Present Progressive Verb Form: *Be + -ing*

The present progressive verb form describes actions in progress at the time of speaking. To form the present progressive, combine *be* with the *-ing* form of the verb.

I *am going* for a walk.
He *is shopping* at the store.
We *are studying* basic nutrition.
They *are talking* to the doctor.

B. Continue to look at the pictures and listen to the story. Then, retell the story to a partner. Help your partner with new vocabulary. Write the new vocabulary next to the pictures.

C. What advice can you give Roberto about his eating habits?

Modals and Expressions of Advice

The following modals and expressions are listed in the order of strength.

Must	Something is a strong necessity. You don't have a choice. Judy broke her leg. She *must* go to the hospital. To be a doctor, you *must* go to medical school.
Have to	Something is a necessity. They have the flu. They *have to* see the doctor. I *have to* take my medicine before I go to sleep.
Should	Something is suggested, but you make the choice. Bill doesn't feel well. He *should* stay in bed. You have a headache. You *should* take an aspirin.
Ought to	Something is suggested, but you make the choice. Bill doesn't feel well. He *ought to* stay in bed. You have a headache. You *ought to* take an aspirin.
Had better	Something is suggested, or something negative may be the result. You *had better* pay your medical bills soon. You *had better* follow the doctor's orders.

In the space provided, write four suggestions.

Example: Roberto had better eat more fruit.

1.

2.

3.

4.

Now, in the space provided, write four sentences telling Roberto what to do. Use the imperative form.

Example: Do not eat high-fat foods.

1.

2.

3.

4.

Review your sentences. Which sentences sound more polite? Which sound more demanding. If you were Roberto, which would you like to hear? Why?

II. The Food Guide Pyramid

The U.S. Department of Agriculture and the U.S. Department of Health and Human Services are governmental organizations. They developed a system. This system helps people with their eating habits. It is called the Food Guide Pyramid. The pyramid can help you choose what to eat each day. It can also help you choose how much to eat. Follow the Food Guide Pyramid to eat a variety of foods. The pyramid will help to keep you healthy.

The Food Guide Pyramid

A Guide to Daily Food Choices

KEY

◘ **Fat** (naturally occurring and added)

▼ **Sugars** (added)

These symbols show fat and added sugars in foods.

Fats, Oils, & Sweets
USE SPARINGLY

Milk, Yogurt, & Cheese Group
2-3 SERVINGS

Benefits: protein, calcium, and vitamins (important for energy, strong bones, and teeth)

Meat, Poultry, Fish, Dry Beans, Eggs, & Nuts Group
2-3 SERVINGS

Benefits: iron and protein (important for energy and strong muscles)

Vegetable Group
3-5 SERVINGS

Benefits: fiber, vitamins A and C, and iron (important for healthy skin, bones, and eyes)

Fruit Group
2-4 SERVINGS

Benefits: Vitamins A and C, fiber (important for healthy bones and eyes)

Bread, Cereal, Rice, & Pasta Group
6-11 SERVINGS

Benefits: carbohydrates (important for energy)

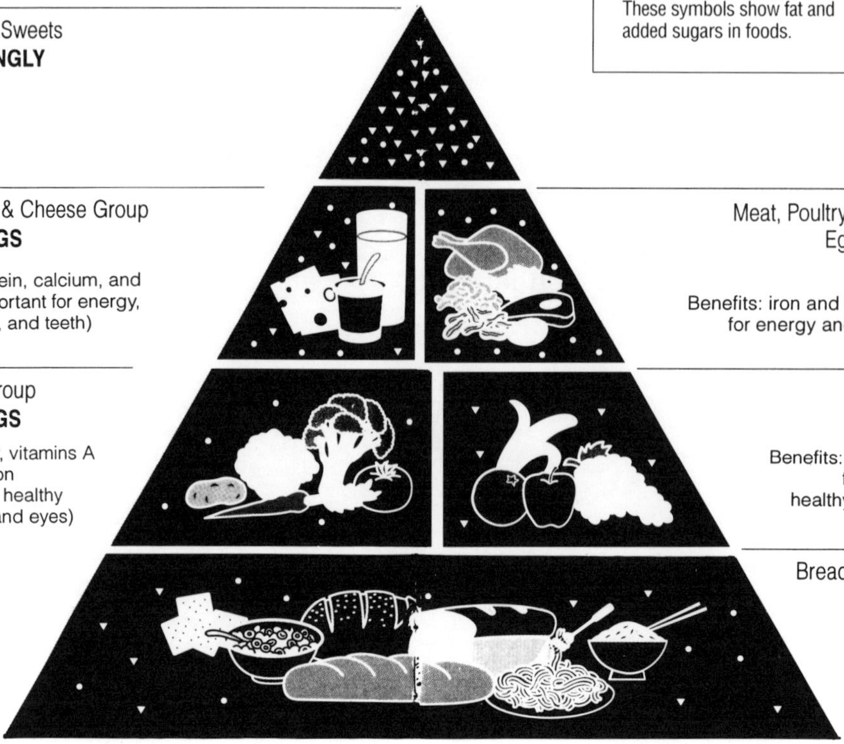

The Food Guide Pyramid, Human Nutrition Information Service, U.S. Department of Agriculture, August 1992.

A. Study the Food Guide Pyramid. Scan for the answers to the following questions.

1. What does ◘ mean?

   What does ▼ mean?

2. Do milk products contain fat?

   Do meat products contain fat?

   How do you know?

3. How many daily servings of fruit should a person have?

4. A person should consume (eat or drink) 3–5 servings of what?

5. We need the most servings from which group?

6. Should a person have more servings of fruit or more of milk?

7. What are the benefits of vegetables?

8. Which foods help build strong bones and teeth?

9. Why do we need carbohydrates?

10. Which foods are good sources of fiber?

B. Study the following list of food items. Each item equals one serving. Decide which food group each item belongs in. Write the letters on the line. An example is shown.

Food Groups

B = Bread Group	ME = Meat Group
F = Fruit Group	MI = Milk Group
V = Vegetable Group	

1.	B	1 slice of bread	5.	______	1 egg
2.	______	1/2 cup of cooked beans	6.	______	1 cup of milk
3.	______	1 banana	7.	______	1/2 cup of vegetables
4.	______	3/4 cup of juice	8.	______	2 large crackers

9. ______ 2 to 3 ounces of cooked lean meat
10. ______ 1/2 cup of cooked rice
11. ______ 1 cup (8 ounces) of yogurt
12. ______ 1/2 cup of cooked pasta
13. ______ 2 to 3 ounces of fish
14. ______ 1 medium apple
15. ______ 1-1/2 ounces of natural cheese

Nouns: Count and Noncount

You can count many food items. For example, you might eat two cookies, a banana, or three crackers for a snack. A count noun has both a singular form (one egg) and a plural form (two eggs). There are some items you cannot count. Items like milk, rice, and pasta are noncount items. Noncount nouns do not have plural forms.

Nouns: Measurement Forms

When you refer to the amount of many food items (both count and noncount nouns), you often use a form of measurement. Measurement forms include *slice, bag, jar, can, package, carton,* and *bunch.* Measurement forms also include a weight or size like *pound (lb.), ounce (oz.), cup (C. or c.), teaspoon (t. or tsp.)* or *tablespoon (T. or Tbl.).*

C. Study the list of food items in Activity B again. Circle all the noncount nouns. Then, begin to make a list of noncount nouns.

Noncount Nouns

D. Match the measurement form and food noun to the appropriate picture.

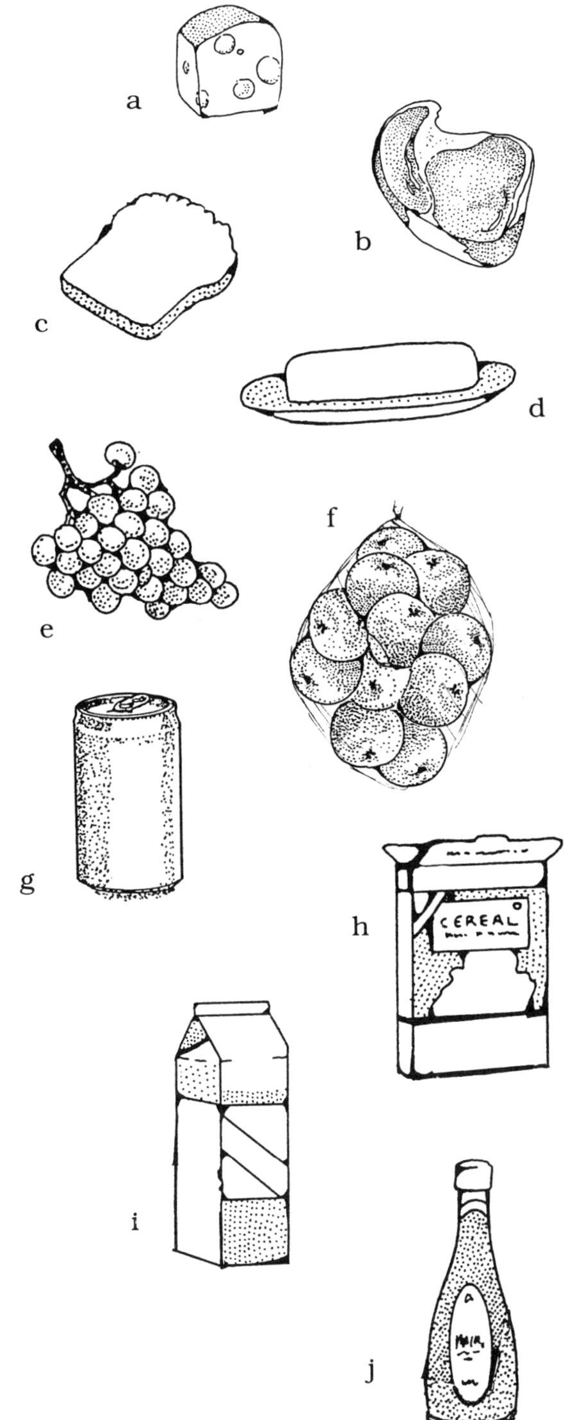

1. ______ bunch of grapes
2. ______ bag of oranges
3. ______ carton of milk
4. ______ stick of butter
5. ______ can of soda
6. ______ pound (lb.) of meat
7. ______ ounce (oz.) of cheese
8. ______ bottle of ketchup
9. ______ slice of bread
10. ______ box of cereal

E. Write your own sentences using the simple past form of the verb and the words that follow. Add any new verbs to your list on page 38. For words you do not know, use your dictionary.

Examples:

cook, cup, rice	I cooked two cups of rice.
buy, bunch, banana	Joan bought a bunch of bananas.

1. open, carton, milk ______________________
2. peel, bag, carrots ______________________
3. eat, bunch, grapes ______________________
4. drink, glass, juice ______________________
5. grate, ounce, cheese ______________________
6. cut, slice, bread ______________________
7. drink, can, soda ______________________
8. measure, teaspoon (tsp.), salt ______________________
9. buy, carton, eggs ______________________
10. cook, box, pasta ______________________

III. Smart Choices and Food Logs

A. Read the following passage.

Roberto wasn't feeling well, so he visited his doctor. "What seems to be the problem?" the doctor asked.

"I am always tired," explained Roberto. "I come home from work and have no energy. I'm very concerned."

The doctor examined and weighed Roberto. He had gained 15 pounds! "Your problem is your weight, Roberto. You had better improve your eating habits," warned Dr. Foster. "You should learn more about the foods you eat."

Dr. Foster explained the Food Guide Pyramid to Roberto. He also gave him a chart of smart food choices. The chart lists the foods a person should eat often, sometimes, and seldom. Finally, Dr. Foster advised Roberto to keep a food log. A food log is a list of what a person eats. Roberto can study his log and make changes in his diet.

B. Dr. Foster gave Roberto several tools to help him develop healthy habits. Match each tool to the *best* definition.

1. ______ Food Guide Pyramid
2. ______ Food Log
3. ______ Smart Choices Chart

a. helps you choose the best foods
b. shows you what you ate
c. tells you the number of servings to eat

C. Look at the chart from Dr. Foster's office and answer the questions that follow.

Smart Choices
From the Office of Dr. Foster

Eat these foods:

	Often	Sometimes	Seldom
Bread	whole grain bread, whole grain cereal, plain popcorn, pasta, brown rice	white bread, white rice, pretzels, crackers	sweetened cereal, muffins, chips
Fruit	fresh fruit	fruit juice, dried fruit	canned fruit in syrup, sweetened juice
Vegetables	fresh vegetables, vegetable juice	frozen vegetables	canned vegetables, french fries
Meat	chicken, turkey, low-fat fish, water-packed tuna, egg whites, tofu	lean beef, lamb, pork, shellfish, nuts	steak, bacon, sausage, oil-packed tuna, hot dogs, luncheon meats, egg yolks

	Often	Sometimes	Seldom
Milk	nonfat milk, low-fat milk, nonfat or low-fat yogurt	low-fat cheese, frozen yogurt	whole milk, whole-milk yogurt, ice cream
Fats, oils, sweets, other	water, tea, spices, nonfat dressings	coffee, low-fat dressings, mayonnaise, mustard	soda, butter, cake, candy, doughnuts, alcoholic beverages

Which should Roberto eat more of?

1. whole grain bread or chips

    ____

2. white rice or brown rice

    ____

3. turkey or lean beef ______________________________

Adverbs of Frequency

Adverbs of frequency tell how often something happens. Examples of adverbs of frequency are *always*, *sometimes*, and *never*. Adverbs of frequency range from *always* (100%) to *never* (0%).

100% - 0%

always often sometimes seldom never

Adverbs of frequency are located

1. before the simple present or simple past verb.
   Roberto never went to the doctor's office.
2. after a modal (or first auxiliary verb).
   You should seldom eat after 9:00 P.M.
3. after the main *be* verb.
   Roberto is often hungry for pizza.
4. before the imperative verb.
   Always eat from the five food groups.

D. Rewrite the sentences, adding the adverb of frequency.

Example:

I eat breakfast at 7 A.M. (always)
I always eat breakfast at 7 A.M.

1. I drink three glasses of milk. (seldom)

2. My mom cooks with lean meat. (often)

3. Alper is sick. (never)

4. Eat bacon or sausage. (seldom)

5. The doctor was very busy. (sometimes)

6. Try to consume a variety of foods. (always)

7. Tamer is dieting. (often)

E. Think about your own eating habits. Write a sentence answering the following. Use an adverb of frequency in your sentence.

How often do you ____________?

Example:
have three servings of milk   I usually have three servings of milk.

1. eat fresh fruit

2. have 6–11 servings of bread

3. drink nonfat or lowfat milk

4. consume 3–5 servings of vegetables

5. eat white rice

6. eat chicken

F. In this activity, you will analyze Roberto's eating habits. First, study the Food Guide Pyramid on page 80. Then, read Roberto's food log. Compare Roberto's food log to the suggested servings.

Monday

Breakfast
- 1 glass of orange juice
- 1 banana
- 2 chocolate doughnuts

Lunch
- 1 hotdog with ketchup
- 1 slice of cheese
- 1 hotdog bun
- 1 bag of potato chips
- 1 can of cola

Dinner
- 2 large pieces of sausage pizza
- 1 small salad
- 1 large cola

Snacks
- 2 oatmeal cookies
- 1 glass of milk

	Suggested Servings	*Roberto's Servings*
Bread	6–11	______
Fruit	2–4	______
Vegetables	3–5	______
Meat	2–3	______
Milk	2–3	______

G. Study the Smart Choices chart on pages 85–86. Roberto does not always choose his food wisely. He could make better food choices. Write three improvements for Roberto.

Examples:
Don't eat doughnuts.
Roberto should eat whole grain cereal with lowfat milk.

1.

2.

3.

H. Is *your* diet a healthy diet? To find out, follow these steps:

Step 1. *Keep a food log.* Make a list of everything you ate yesterday. Include meals and snacks. Be sure to use an appropriate form of measurement (e.g., one slice of white bread).

Food Log
Date: ______________________________
Breakfast
Lunch
Dinner
Snacks

Step 2. *Study the Food Guide Pyramid.* Compare your food log with the suggested servings. Did you have the correct number of servings from the five major food groups?

	Suggested Servings	*Your Servings*
Bread	6–11	______
Fruit	2–4	______
Vegetables	3–5	______
Meat	2–3	______
Milk	2–3	______

Step 3. *Study the Smart Choices chart.* Compare what you ate to the chart. Write some healthy changes on your food log.

Step 4. *Develop a plan.* Make a list of ways to improve your daily eating habits.

Examples:

Add an extra serving of fruit each day.
I ought to eat whole grain bread instead of white bread.

1.

2.

3.

Step 5. *Write a paragraph.* Write a paragraph that describes your current eating habits and explains your plan for improvement. Use future verb forms to describe what you will do.

Future Verb Forms: *Will* and *Be Going To*

To show future time, use *will* + simple verb form.

I	will	eat	more fruit.
He	will	drink	less soda.
They	will	choose	wheat bread.

To show a prior future plan, use *be going to* + simple verb form.

She	is going to	cook	more chicken.
They	are going to	consume	less red meat.
We	are going to	drink	a lot of water.

IV. Reading Food Labels

By law, companies must include certain information on their food labels. The information helps you choose the best food for your needs. This information includes the name of the product. It also includes the ingredients and nutrients (protein, calcium) in the product.

A. In the next activity, you will read the passage "Nutrition Facts." But first, study the italicized words in the sentences. Determine the meaning of these words.

A *brand* is the company's product name.
Nutrients help provide healthy life and growth.
Calories are the amount of food energy.
Ingredients are the things in the food product.
Labels explain what the products are.
A *serving* is the amount of food for one person.

Now, use the italicized words in the following sentences.

1. The average woman should eat about 1,800 ________________ each day.
2. When a famous person advertises a certain ________________, the product often sells better.

3. Always eat different foods each day. This way, you will get all of the ____________________ your body needs to stay healthy.
4. I did not make enough dessert, so each guest can have only one ____________________ of cake.
5. Read all ________________ carefully before you buy products.
6. Do we have all of the ____________________ (eggs, flour, butter) to make a cake?

B. You should now understand the vocabulary. Read the passage and circle the words you learned in Activity A.

Nutrition Facts

When you eat the right foods, you enjoy better health. You also reduce (lower) your chances of getting sick. Learn to read the labels of foods you eat. Labels can help you make smart food choices. Most labels contain Nutrition Facts. Nutrition Facts are accurate and easy to understand. They can tell you the following information:

a. *Servings.* Each label includes the serving size and the number of servings in the package. Serving sizes for similar foods must be the same. This makes it easy to compare different brands (company products). For example, similar brands of cereal must consider a serving to equal 1 ounce.
b. *Calories.* Calories provide energy. Too many calories make you overweight. Too few calories make you underweight. The number of calories for each serving is written on the label. In addition, the number of calories from fat is also provided. Read Nutrition Facts to help you limit your fat intake. Fat should be less than 30 percent of your total calories.
c. *Daily Values.* Important nutrients are listed under Daily Values. These nutrients include total fat, cholesterol, sodium (salt), total carbohydrate, and protein. The labels also list the percentage of vitamins A and C, calcium, and iron.
d. *Ingredients.* Ingredients are listed in the order of amount. The item listed first has the largest amount. The item listed last has the smallest amount.

C. Use the information in "Nutrition Facts" to identify the information on this label. On each line, write the correct vocabulary term.

1. ______________________________

2. ______________________________

3. ______________________________

4. ______________________________

5. ______________________________

serving size
brand name
calories
daily values
ingredients

Keebler

Wheatables®

Wheat Snack Crackers

Nutrition Facts

Serving Size 26 crackers (30g)
Servings Per Container about 7

Amount Per Serving	
Calories 150	Calories from Fat 60
	% Daily Value*
Total Fat 7g	**11%**
Saturated Fat 2g	**10%**
Cholesterol 0mg	**0%**
Sodium 320mg	**13%**
Total Carbohydrate 18g	**6%**
Dietary Fiber 1g	**4%**
Sugars 2g	
Protein 3g	

Vitamin A 0% •	Vitamin C 0%
Calcium 0% •	Iron 6%

*Percent Daily Values are based on a 2,000 calorie diet. Your daily values may be higher or lower depending on your calorie needs:

	Calories:	2,000	2,500
Total Fat	Less than	65g	80g
Sat Fat	Less than	20g	25g
Cholesterol	Less than	300mg	300mg
Sodium	Less than	2,400mg	2,400mg
Total Carbohydrate		300g	375g
Dietary Fiber		25g	30g

INGREDIENTS: ENRICHED FLOUR [WHEAT FLOUR, NIACIN, REDUCED IRON, THIAMINE MONONITRATE (VITAMIN B1) AND RIBOFLAVIN (VITAMIN B2)], VEGETABLE SHORTENING (PARTIALLY HYDROGENATED SOYBEAN AND/OR COTTONSEED OILS), DEHYDRATED POTATOES, STEAMED CRUSHED WHEAT, SALT, SUGAR, DEFATTED WHEAT GERM, CORN SYRUP, MALT, ONION POWDER, MONOSODIUM GLUTAMATE, SOY LECITHIN, SODIUM BICARBONATE, SPICE, NATURAL FLAVOR.

Every product from Keebler is meant to be Uncommonly Good. Should you have reason to write us regarding this product, please send your comments, along with top flap of box with stamped-in code to: Keebler Company, Consumer Relations, 1 Hollow Tree Lane, Elmhurst, IL 60126.

ELMHURST, ILLINOIS 60126
REG. PENNA. DEPT. AGR. MADE IN U.S.A.

D. Now, answer the questions about the passage "Nutrition Facts" from page 92.

1. Why is it easy to compare different brands?

2. What happens if you do not get enough calories?

Keebler label courtesy of the Keebler Company.

3. How much fat should a person consume each day?

4. How are ingredients listed on a label?

E. Read the questions and scan the labels to find the information. Write answers to the questions on page 96.

Nutrition Facts
Serving Size 1/2 cup (125g)
Servings Per Container approx. 3 1/2
Amount Per Serving
Calories 60 Calories from Fat 0
% Daily Value*
Total Fat 0g 0%
Saturated Fat 0g 0%
Cholesterol 0mg 0%
Sodium 360mg 15%
Total Carbohydrate 11g 4%
Dietary Fiber 4g 16%
Sugars 6g
Protein 3g
Vitamin A 4% • Vitamin C 30%
Calcium 2% • Iron 8%
*Percent Daily Values are based on a 2,000 calorie diet.
INGREDIENTS: PEAS, WATER, SUGAR, SALT
©1989 DISTRIBUTED BY DEL MONTE FOODS SAN FRANCISCO, CA 94105 PACKED IN U.S.A.
WHEN WRITING TO US, COPY THE CODE FROM THE END OF THE CAN.
Vegetables may reduce your risk of some types of cancer because they are low in fat and may contain Vitamin A, Vitamin C, or dietary fiber. DEL MONTE® Sweet Peas are an excellent source of Vitamin C and a good source of dietary fiber. Include DEL MONTE Sweet Peas in your diet for better health!
Microwave: Empty contents into microwavable dish; cover; heat 3 minutes. Season to taste; serve.
*WT. OF PEAS (9 1/4 OZ.) BEFORE ADDITION OF LIQUID NECESSARY FOR PROCESSING
0 24000 16308 4
PLEASE RECYCLE

AMERICA'S ★CHOICE★ SKIM MILK
GRADE A • PASTEURIZED • HOMOGENIZED • VITAMIN A & D
Nutrition Facts
Serving Size 1 cup (240 mL)
Servings 16
Calories 90
Fat Cal. 10
*Percent Daily Values (DV) are based on a 2,000 calorie diet.
Amount/serving %DV* Amount/serving %DV*
Total Fat 1g 2% Total Carb. 12g 4%
Sat. Fat 0.5g 3% Fiber 0g 0%
Cholest. 5mg 2% Sugars 11g
Sodium 125mg 5% Protein 8g
Vitamin A 10% • Vitamin C 4% • Calcium 30%
Iron 0% • Vitamin D 25% • Phosphorus 25%
INGREDIENTS: SKIM MILK, VITAMIN A PALMITATE AND VITAMIN D3.
DISTRIBUTED BY COMPASS FOODS, MONTVALE, NJ 07645
PROCESSED AT PLANT STAMPED BELOW • KEEP REFRIGERATED
LESS THAN 1/2% MILKFAT.
1 GAL (3.78L)
SELL BY:
MAY 14

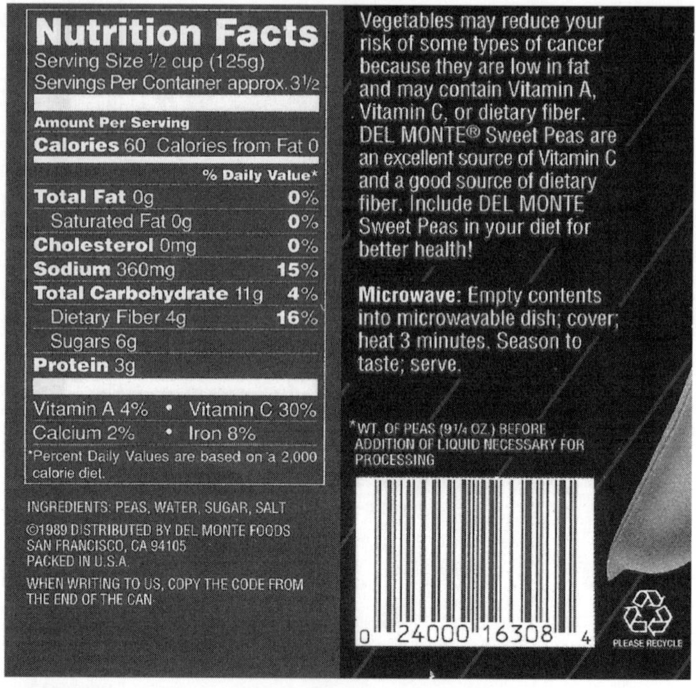

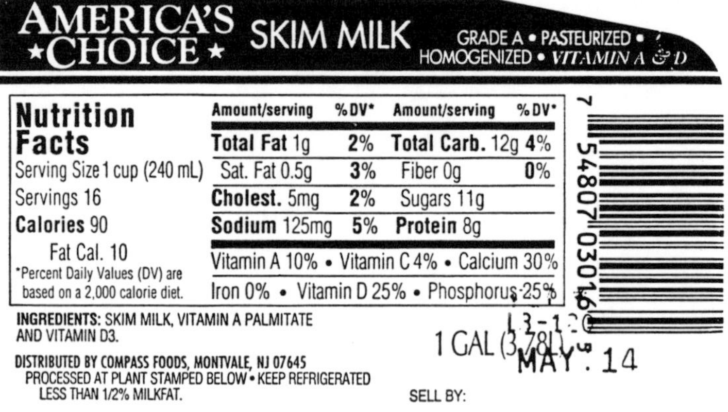

Pea label courtesy of Del Monte Foods.
Milk label courtesy of The Great Atlantic & Pacific Tea Company. Copyright The Great Atlantic & Pacific Tea Company, Inc., the parent company of Compass Foods, Inc.

Nutrition Facts

Serving Size 1 oz. (28g/About 6 chips)
Servings Per Container 20

Amount Per Serving

Calories 130	Calories from Fat 50
	% Daily Value*
Total Fat 6g	**9%**
Saturated Fat 1g	**5%**
Cholesterol 0mg	**0%**
Sodium 80mg	**3%**
Total Carbohydrate 19g	**6%**
Dietary Fiber 1g	**5%**
Sugars 0g	
Protein 2g	

Vitamin A 0%	•	Vitamin C 0%
Calcium 4%	•	Iron 0%

* Percent Daily Values are based on a 2,000 calorie diet. Your daily values may be higher or lower depending on your calorie needs:

	Calories:	2,000	2,500
Total Fat	Less than	65g	80g
Sat Fat	Less than	20g	25g
Cholesterol	Less than	300mg	300mg
Sodium	Less than	2,400mg	2,400mg
Total Carbohydrate		300g	375g
Dietary Fiber		25g	30g

Calories per gram:
Fat 9 • Carbohydrate 4 • Protein 4

INGREDIENTS: WHITE CORN, VEGETABLE OIL (CONTAINS ONE OR MORE OF THE FOLLOWING: CANOLA, CORN, OR PARTIALLY HYDROGENATED (CANOLA OR SOYBEAN) OIL), AND SALT.

NO PRESERVATIVES.

FRITO-LAY, INC.
DALLAS, TEXAS 75235-5224
©RECOT, INC., 1990

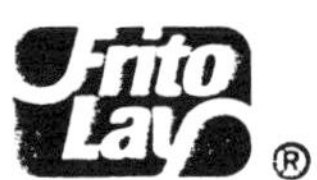

Frito-Lay label courtesy of Frito-Lay, Inc.

Nutrition Facts
Serving Size 1 bagel (80g)
Servings Per Container 5

Amount Per Serving	
Calories 210	Calories from Fat 15
	% Daily Value*
Total Fat 1.5g	**3%**
Saturated Fat 0g	**0%**
Cholesterol 0mg	**0%**
Sodium 270mg	**11%**
Total Carbohydrate 41g	**14%**
Dietary Fiber 2g	**10%**
Sugars 4g	
Protein 8g	
Vitamin A 0% • Vitamin C 2%	
Calcium 6% • Iron 15%	

*Percent Daily Values are based on a 2,000 calorie diet. Your daily values may be higher or lower depending on your calorie needs:

	Calories:	2,000	2,500
Total Fat	Less than	65g	80g
Sat Fat	Less than	20g	25g
Cholesterol	Less than	300mg	300mg
Sodium	Less than	2,400mg	2,400mg
Total Carbohydrate		300g	375g
Dietary Fiber		25g	30g

Ingredients:
High Gluten Flour, Whole Wheat Flour, Water, Honey, Malt, Brown Sugar, Salt, Bran, Vegetable Oil, Yeast, Calcium Propionate, Potassium Sorbate (preserves freshness), Rice Flour.

1. What foods are these labels from?

2. Two labels contain brand names. What are the brand names of these foods?

3. List the ingredients in a bagel.

4. Which product contains no fat?

Bagel label courtesy of Uncle B's Bakery, Ellsworth, Iowa.

5. How many servings are in the container of milk?

6. How many calories are in one serving of chips?

7. How many grams of protein are in a serving of milk?

8. Which of these foods contains the most calories per serving?

9. How many calories come from fat in a serving of chips?
   Is this a high-fat food?

10. Which of these foods contains the highest total fat content per serving?

V. Fast Foods

Fast food restaurants and cafeterias are very popular in the United States. It is quick and easy to get a meal in these places. Unfortunately, fast foods are usually high in sodium, fat, and calories. But it is possible to buy healthy foods in fast food restaurants or cafeterias. Some menu choices are better than others.

A. Read the passage about Roberto and Peri. They just finished their English class and are now going to the cafeteria.

   "I am starving!" exclaimed Roberto. "I didn't have time for lunch today. I could eat three hamburgers right now!" As soon as Roberto said this, he remembered his doctor's advice. Roberto told Peri about his visit to the doctor. "I gained 15 pounds, Peri. I have little energy and my jeans are so tight!" Peri worked many hours at the movie theater and she studied English too. But she always seemed to have energy. "How do you stay healthy, Peri?" Roberto asked. "You always look good."

"Well," began Peri. "When I first moved here, it was difficult. I had to learn which foods were healthy and which foods were not. I used to think American food was not good, but now I know I can make healthy choices. Even fast food restaurants and cafeterias have items that are good for you."

By this time, Roberto and Peri were at the cafeteria. It was crowded with people talking and laughing. Peri continued, "If you want, I'll explain the best choices, Roberto." "That would be great!" exclaimed Roberto.

B. Answer the following questions about the passage.

1. Why was Roberto very hungry?

2. Where does Peri work?

3. How does Peri stay healthy?

4. What does Peri think of American food?

C. Peri said that it is possible to order healthy foods in fast food restaurants and cafeterias. She said that some menu choices are better than others. Read Peri's suggestions and make a list of any words you do not understand. Discuss the meanings with a classmate and your teacher.

Peri's Suggestions

Let's look at the salad bar. Nowadays, most restaurants offer salad bars. Salad bars contain fresh vegetables and salads like pasta and potato salads. First, choose fresh vegetables like lettuce, carrots, and tomatoes. Do not choose pasta or potato salads. They contain extra fat. Second, be careful of bacon, cheese, and sunflower seeds. These items can change a lowfat, healthy salad into a high-fat one. Toppings like beans or peas are better. Finally, use a small amount of dressing. Dressings in restaurants are often high in calories and sodium.

Now let's look at a menu. When you choose foods from a menu, look for key words. First, *broiled, grilled,* or *baked* foods are better than *fried* foods. For example, eat a baked potato, not french fries. Instead of a fried chicken sandwich, order a grilled chicken sandwich. Second, order *steamed* or *fresh* vegetables, not *buttered* or *creamed* vegetables. Third, plain foods are the best. For example, a piece of lean chicken is better than chicken and gravy. Foods in sauces or gravy contain a lot of fat, calories, and salt.

Small changes can help you to improve your health. For example, order vegetable or cheese pizza instead of pepperoni or sausage pizza. Order sandwiches with whole grain bread, not white bread. Pretzels or plain popcorn is better than potato chips. Often order juice or low fat milk. Rarely order soda or milkshakes. Small changes like these can put you in the right direction toward more healthy eating habits.

D. Reread "Peri's Suggestions" and complete the chart.

	Choose	Do not choose
Salad bar items		
Menu items		
Small changes		

E. Study the following menu.

Donna's Deli

Salad Bar

The salad bar includes lettuce and dressing. Choose five additional ingredients: peas, carrots, cheese, mushrooms, green onions, sunflower seeds, tomatoes, green pepper, beans, and bacon.

small	$3.25
large	$4.25

Sandwiches

Sandwiches are served with your choice of whole grain or white bread. In addition, choose two of the following ingredients: tomato slices, lettuce, cheese, Donna's homemade sauce, pickles, and onion.

Grilled chicken	$4.59
Fried chicken	4.35
Tuna salad	4.25
Hamburger	3.75
Steak	6.49

Pizza

Choose two of the following ingredients: tomatoes, sausage, pepperoni, onion, black olives, green pepper, shrimp, hamburger, and mushrooms.

Per slice	$2.36

Vegetables

French fries	$1.50
Baked potato	1.50
Steamed vegetables	1.25
Creamed corn	1.09

Beverages

Coffee	.59
Decaf	.59
Hot tea	.59
Iced tea	.89
Soft drinks	.99
Cola, diet cola, root beer	
Lowfat milk	.75
Milkshakes	1.49
Vanilla, chocolate, strawberry	
Fruit juices	1.25
Apple, orange, cranberry	

Desserts

Ice cream	$1.39
Frozen yogurt	1.39
Fresh fruit	1.50
Apple pie	1.89
Cheesecake	2.25

F. Using the information from the chart in Activity D, select a healthy meal from the menu. Write your selections in the space below.

Chapter 7

Physical Fitness

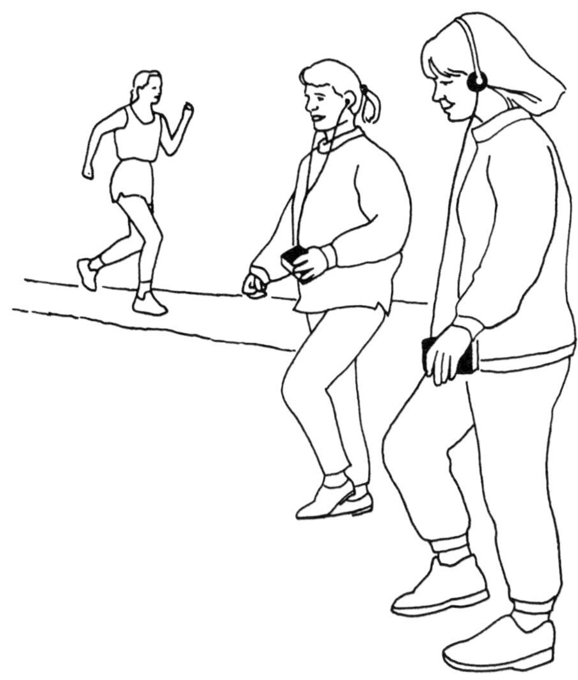

A Look Behind/A Look Ahead

In chapter 6, you studied the importance of healthy eating. The right foods can give you the energy for your busy life.

In addition, physical activity is important. There are many benefits to exercise. Two benefits are an increase in your energy level and a decrease in your stress level. Chapter 7 explains how to keep your interest in exercise. It also discusses the options available to you.

To the Student

After completing this chapter, you will understand

1. how to keep your interest in exercise, and
2. the options that may be available to you.

Vocabulary Development

Put a check (✓) on the line to the left of all the words you understand. Write the part of speech to the right. The first two are done for you. Then, finish this chapter and return to this list. Check or write in all new words you learned. Review these words often!

___ exercise ___n/v___	___ community ______	___ motivation ______
___ injury ___n___	___ team ______	___ fitness ______
___ tennis ______	___ aerobics ______	___ golf ______
___ baseball ______	___ energy ______	___ swimming ______
___ recreational ______	___ weight lifting ______	___ goal ______
______	______	______
______	______	______
______	______	______
______	______	______

I. Maintaining Fitness Motivation

A. With another student, talk about the following questions.

1. How often do you exercise?
2. What physical activities do you usually do (walk, swim, cycle, lift weights, run/jog, play a team sport, etc.)?
3. How has your physical activity changed since you moved to this country?

B. Read the following passage.

Hundreds of people begin an exercise program every year. But before long, many of those people stop exercising. They go back to their old habits. These people have many reasons for returning to their old ways. Two popular excuses are "Exercise is boring" and "I don't have time." How can a busy person stay motivated? Following are several suggestions.

1. People make appointments to see the dentist or to get a haircut. They write meeting times in their calendars. Physical activity is important, too. Make "an appointment" to exercise.
2. Exercise for 15 minutes and gradually increase your activity. This will help to prevent injuries or soreness.
3. When you meet your exercise goal, do something special. Go to the movies or buy an inexpensive "gift."
4. Do something you really enjoy. If you like to be with people, join a team. If you like nature, go for a walk.
5. Exercise with a partner. You can encourage and motivate each other. You can have fun, too.
6. Walk one day and swim the next. Play ball with some friends and then go for a bike ride. Try a variety of activities.

C. Read Activity B again and decide what the main idea is for each suggestion. Write a title on the line that explains each main idea. Number one has been done for you.

> Topic Sentence
>
> A paragraph is usually about one topic. Each paragraph has a sentence that tells the topic (the main idea) of the paragraph. It is called the topic sentence. The topic sentence is often the first or the last sentence in a paragraph. The other sentences give details about the topic sentence.

1. Schedule Exercise Time

2. ______________________________

3. ______________________________

4. ______________________________

5. ______________________________

6. ______________________________

D. For each suggestion in Activity B, locate and underline the topic sentence. Check to be sure your title is similar to the topic sentence.

E. With your classmates, decide the order of importance for the six suggestions. What is the best way to stay motivated with an exercise program? For example, is it more important to exercise with a partner or to try a variety of activities? Once you agree, write the order here:

1. ______
2. ______
3. ______
4. ______
5. ______
6. ______

F. Do you exercise regularly? Is a regular exercise plan something you wish to follow? With your classmates, decide on three additional things a person could do to stay motivated. On a piece of paper, write a short paragraph for each idea and underline your topic sentence. Then, provide a title for each paragraph. An example is provided.

Example:

SET SMALL GOALS. You should plan to exercise two or three times this week. Then, make a new plan for next week.

II. The Community Recreational Center

A. Scan the following passage in Activity B to put the events in the correct order. Do not read the entire passage. Read for the appropriate information. The first one is done for you.

According to the story, Roberto ________________________.

________ walked for exercise

________ went to his doctor's office

___1___ gained weight

________ made plans to visit the community recreational center

________ had more energy

B. Now, read the passage carefully.

Approximately three months ago, Roberto visited his doctor. He told the doctor that his eating habits were poor. He was overweight, and he was always tired. His low energy level made it difficult to work and study. After Roberto talked with his doctor, he decided to do something. He decided to get in shape.

Roberto started slowly. He set small goals. Every night before dinner, he walked for 20 minutes. At first, it was very difficult. Sometimes, he had an excuse: "I'm too tired tonight. I'll exercise tomorrow." But Roberto didn't give up. The next day, he was out walking again.

In addition to exercise, Roberto watched what he ate. Sometimes, he ate a cookie or some ice cream, but he was careful not to eat too much. He remembered something his doctor told him: "No food is bad food. It is the amount that is important." Soon, Roberto began to see and feel a difference. His clothes fit better, his energy level increased, and he felt better about himself.

One night while Roberto was walking, he saw his neighbor, Jill. "Hi, Jill! How are you?"

"I'm fine, Roberto. I've seen you walking a lot lately. That's great! You should visit the community recreational center sometime. There are a variety of activities. I'm on a baseball team that plays every Saturday. It's a lot of fun, you get to meet people, and it's inexpensive."

"That sounds interesting. Does the center have tennis?"

"Yes, it sure does. It has practically everything."

Jill and Roberto talked for a while about the local community center and made plans to meet there Thursday night. As Roberto finished his walk, he thought about the changes of the last three months.

C. Decide whether these sentences are true (T) or false (F). Then, rewrite the false sentences to make them true.

Example:

doctor

__F__ Roberto visited his ~~dentist~~.

______ 1. Every morning, Roberto walked for 20 minutes.

______ 2. Roberto ate no desserts on his diet.

______ 3. Roberto had more energy, and he felt better.

______ 4. Roberto didn't like to walk, so he joined the community center.

______ 5. The community recreational center is free.

______ 6. Jill plays baseball at the community center.

D. Answer the following questions. Try to answer without looking at the passage.

1. Why did Roberto see his doctor?

2. What did Roberto do to get in shape?

3. What happened after Roberto changed his habits?

4. What can you do at a community center?

E. At the community recreational center, Roberto found a chart of activities. He studied the chart before he made any decisions. With your partner, complete the recreational chart. One person should be Partner A and the other, Partner B (Partner B's chart is in appendix A, page 112). Do not look at each other's chart! Take turns asking for information, and write it in the boxes.

> Review: Providing and Receiving Information
>
> You may need to ask your partner to spell or repeat words. You can ask: "How do you spell that?" "Can you repeat that?" When you spell a word, follow this pattern: "The contact person is Paco. That's P as in *park*, A, C as in *cat*, O."

Partner A

Community Recreational Center					
Activity	Equipment Needed	Meeting Times	Contact Person	Phone Number	Membership Fee
Tennis		MWF 6–8 P.M.	Paco		$27.50
Weight lifting			Hussein	881-1930	$15.00
Aerobics	3-pound weights	M–F 6–8:30 P.M.			$20.00
Swimming		MWThF 6:45–8:30 P.M.		608-3581	$22.00
	glove bat	Sat. 2–5:30 P.M.	Rob	753-4511	$15.50
	clubs balls	TTh 3–5:15 P.M. Sun, 9–12	Irit	651-3650	

F. Using the chart, answer the following questions. Use short answers.

1. When can you swim at the community center?

2. How much does it cost to play tennis?

3. Who should you call about joining aerobics? What is her phone number?

4. What activity requires no equipment?

5. What activity has the most expensive membership fee?

6. What equipment is needed for baseball?

G. Interview a classmate about an exercise or sport that he or she knows about.

1. What is the exercise or sport called?

2. What equipment or clothing is needed?

3. How many players are required?

4. What are some of the rules of the exercise or sport?

5. How much time is required to play the exercise or sport?

6. What special skills are required to play?

7. Why do you like this activity?

H. Most cities have a local community center. Write three questions you could ask a center about its activities. Then, find your local community center in the phone book. Call the center and write the answers to your questions.

Questions

1.

2.

3.

Answers

1.

2.

3.

I. Write a paragraph about an exercise or sport. Use the information from your interview and your phone call. When you are done, check the sentence structure and verb tense in each sentence.

Appendix A

Partner B

Community Recreational Center					
Activity	Equipment Needed	Meeting Times	Contact Person	Phone Number	Member-ship Fee
Tennis	racket balls	MWF 6–8 P.M.		753-8121	$27.50
Weight lift-ing		Daily 4–5 P.M.	Hussein	881-1930	
	3-pound weights	M–F 6–8:30 P.M.	Jackie	651-2942	
Swimming	swimsuit towel		Ruth	608-3581	
Baseball		Sat. 2–5:30 P.M.			$15.50
Golf	clubs balls	TTh 3–5:15 P.M. Sun, 9–12	Irit		$30.50

Chapter 8

Managing Stress

Check (✓) any event that happened to you in the last year. The more events you check, the more stress you have in your life and the more you need to know about handling stress.

Stressful Events

_______ Divorce
_______ Marriage
_______ Death of close family member
_______ Major illness or injury
_______ Major health change of family member
_______ Pregnancy
_______ Change in jobs
_______ Change in job responsibilities
_______ Big personal achievement
_______ Starting or finishing school
_______ Change in living location
_______ Change in recreational activities
_______ Change in sleeping habits
_______ Change in eating habits
_______ Vacation

A Look Behind/A Look Ahead

Chapter 7 discussed ways to maintain your fitness motivation. Regular exercise can improve your health and can help you lose or maintain your weight. It can also help you reduce stress.

Chapter 8 discusses the signs and symptoms of stress. It also provides suggestions for handling stress, including through relaxation.

To the Student

After completing this chapter, you will

1. know the signs and symptoms of stress,
2. understand how to handle stress, and
3. understand how to use relaxation techniques.

Vocabulary Development

Put a check (✓) on the line next to all the words you understand. Finish this chapter and return to this list. Check or write in all new words you learned.

__ signs	__ stress	__ relaxation
__ physical	__ mental	__ emotional
__ tension	__ concentration	__ depression
__ insomnia	__ boredom	__ breathe
__ inhale	__ exhale	__ tense
________	________	________
________	________	________
________	________	________
________	________	________

I. Signs of Stress

A. With a classmate, discuss the following.

1. What is stress?
2. What causes stress?
3. What are the symptoms of stress?
4. What do you do to relax?

B. Scan the passage in Activity C to decide whether these sentences are true (T) or false (F). Read to find the information needed. Do not read all of the passage. Then, correct the false sentences to make them true.

Example:

can
__F__ Stress ~~cannot~~ seriously affect your health.

_______ 1. It is best to have no stress in your life.

_______ 2. Only unhappy or negative situations cause stress.

_______ 3. Giving a speech may be relaxing to one person and stressful to another.

_______ 4. Dr. Hans Selye is a stress expert.

_______ 5. Headaches, diarrhea, and backaches are common emotional signs of stress.

_______ 6. Shopping a lot may be a sign of stress.

C. Now, read the passage carefully.

Managing Stress

You need stress in your life! Does that surprise you? Without stress, life would be dull and unexciting. Too much stress, however, can seriously affect your physical and mental health.

Stress is with us all the time. A major event like a marriage or the loss of a job can cause stress. An exam, traffic, poor eating habits, or even a new friendship can cause stress, too. It is very personal. One person may think an activity is relaxing; another person may think the same activity is stressful. Our reactions to a situation or event cause stress.

Hans Selye, M.D., an expert in the field, defined stress as the body's response to a demand. You need to learn how your body responds to demands. You need to know the early signs of stress. Then, you can learn to control it. Some stress is good, but a lot of stress can be harmful.

Common physical signs of stress include headaches, muscle tension, low back pain, stomach pains, diarrhea, constipation, frequent illness, and weight loss or gain. Common emotional signs include worrying, loss of concentration, depression, and crying. In addition, your behavior may change. You may overeat, smoke, spend money, or avoid people.

Source: Adapted from *Plain Talk About . . . Handling Stress,* Lous E. Kopolow, M.D., U.S. Department of Health and Human Services, Public Health Service Alcohol, Drug Abuse, and Mental Health Administration, National Institute of Mental Health Office of Scientific Information, 1991.

D. Stress is a personal reaction. Your classmates may have very different opinions about situations. One person may enjoy driving in traffic, but another person may find it very stressful.

The Simple Present: Yes/No Question Forms

Do/Does	*Subject*	*Verb*	*Response*
Do	you	like to drive in traffic?	Yes, I do. Yes, I like to drive in traffic. No, I don't. No, I don't like to drive in traffic.
Does	she	dislike loud music?	Yes, she does. Yes, she dislikes loud music. No, she doesn't. No, she doesn't dislike loud music. No, she likes loud music.

What is stressful for your classmates? Find someone in your class to ask each of the following situations or events. Use the correct question format. When you answer a question, use a complete sentence.

Example:

Question: Do you like to meet new people?
Response: (Yes, I do.) Yes, I do like to meet new people.
(No, I don't.) No, I don't like to meet new people.

Find someone who:

Situation/event	Name
1. does not like to meet new people	
2. enjoys listening to loud music	
3. likes to give speeches	
4. enjoys being in a crowd of people	
5. hates driving in heavy traffic	
6. dislikes going to unfamiliar places alone	
7. doesn't mind visiting the dentist	
8. likes to plan and give parties	
9. dislikes taking exams	
10. finds shopping to be very stressful	

E. It is important to recognize the signs and symptoms of stress. Then, you can begin to handle the stress appropriately. Decide whether each of the following is a physical or an emotional sign of stress. Write it under the correct column.

headache
constipation
difficulty concentrating
confusion
undereating
diarrhea
back pain
boredom
chain smoking
skin problems
insomnia
depression
stomachache
anger
crying
the flu
muscle tension
overeating
worrying

Physical	*Emotional*

F. Write a paragraph describing a situation that was very stressful for you. What signs of stress did you have? What did you do about the situation?

II. Handling Stress

A. Read the passage.

We can't live completely without stress, but we can learn to handle and prevent too much stress. Here are some healthy ways to handle stress. You might have additional ideas.

1. When you are nervous, angry, or upset, you should exercise. Running, walking, playing tennis, or working in your garden are just some of the activities you might try. Regular exercise is important for reducing stress.
2. Talk to someone about your concerns and worries. Ask a friend, family member, teacher, or counselor to help you with your problems. If you have a serious problem, you might go to a psychologist, psychiatrist, or mental health counselor.

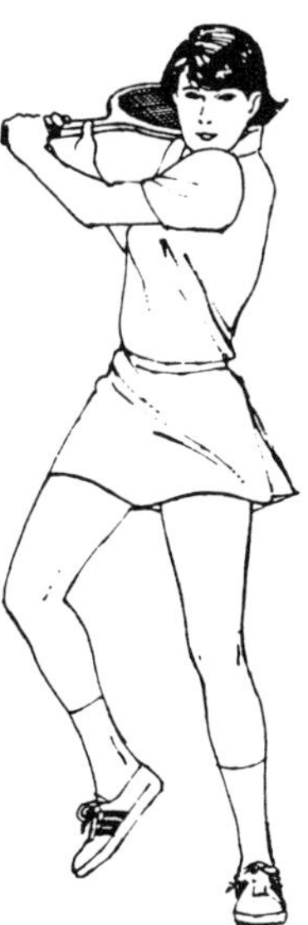

3. Be good to yourself. Get enough rest every day and eat from the basic food groups. Sleep and the right food will help you handle stressful situations.
4. Being alone can make you feel sad, bored, or lonely. Join a neighborhood club or volunteer organization. Get involved in the world and the people around you.
5. Make a list of what you need to do. Then, do one task at a time. Check off each task when you complete it. Do the most important ones first.
6. Prescription and over-the-counter drugs do not remove the cause of stress. Sometimes, they can add to the problems of stress. Take medications only with a doctor's advice.
7. The best way to avoid stress is to relax. Learn to breathe slowly and smoothly. For a while, don't worry about time, problems, or work. Find activities you enjoy. Focus on relaxation, enjoyment, and health.

There are many ways to handle stress. Find ways that work for you.

Source: Adapted from *Plain Talk About . . . Handling Stress*, Lous E. Kopolow, M.D., U.S. Department of Health and Human Services, Public Health Service Alcohol, Drug Abuse, and Mental Health Administration, National Institute of Mental Health Office of Scientific Information, 1991.

B. Read the passage in Activity A again and decide what the main idea is for each numbered paragraph. Write a title below that explains the main idea of the paragraph. The first one is done for you.

1. Try Physical Activity
2. ______________________________
3. ______________________________
4. ______________________________
5. ______________________________
6. ______________________________
7. ______________________________

C. Read and discuss the following situations with your classmates. What other reactions might you have? Together, decide how to reduce your stress. Write your ideas in the space provided.

Situation 1

You will be attending a friend's party this weekend. You know no one but your friend. How will you feel before and during the party? Write three reactions.

Examples:

My muscles will be tense.
I will overeat at the party.

1. ______________________________
2. ______________________________
3. ______________________________

What can you do to reduce the stress?

Situation 2

You are stuck in traffic and are late for an appointment. How will you react? Write three reactions.

Examples:

I will be angry.
I will be worried.

1. ____________________
2. ____________________
3. ____________________

How can you reduce the stress?

Situation 3

You have a final exam next Wednesday morning. You need a high score to pass the course. How will you feel before and during the exam? Write three reactions.

Examples:

I will not be able to concentrate.
I will have diarrhea.

1. ____________________
2. ____________________
3. ____________________

What can you do to reduce the stress?

III. Relaxation

A. Read the passage.

Relaxation is an important part of a healthy lifestyle. Relaxation can greatly reduce your stress level. One way to relax is through deep breathing. Another is through progressive relaxation. With deep breathing, you concentrate on your breathing and forget about your problems or concerns. This is a quick and easy way to reduce stress. In progressive relaxation, you concentrate on the muscles in your body. You tense and then relax those muscles. The more you practice progressive relaxation, the better you get at learning to relax.

B. Look at the pictures. Then, with a classmate, answer the questions.

1. To reduce stress, what does the woman do first?

2. What does she do second?

3. What does she do next?

4. Finally, what does she do?

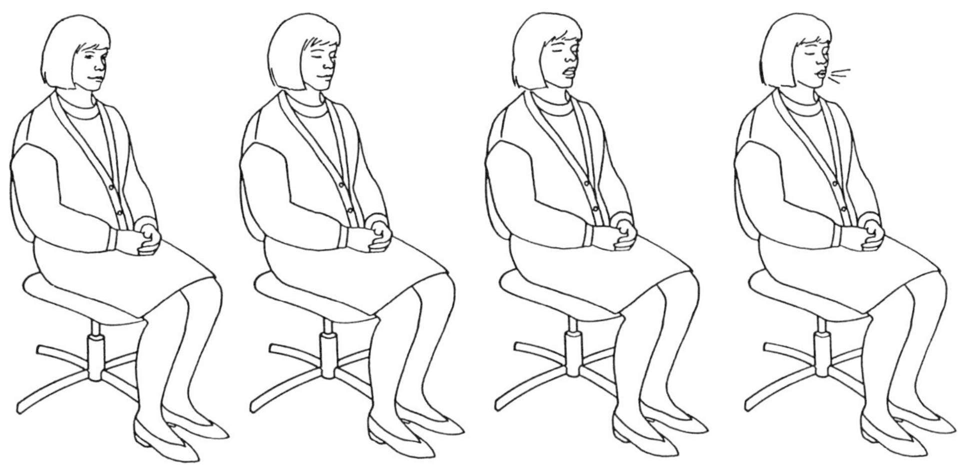

C. Read the paragraph "Deep Breathing". Compare the steps in the paragraph to your answers in Activity B.

Deep Breathing

Deep breathing is a quick and easy way to reduce stress. First, sit up in your chair. Your feet should be on the floor. Your hands should be in your lap. Second, close your eyes. Next, slowly take a deep breath (inhale) and hold for five seconds. Finally, slowly release your breath (exhale) through your mouth. Repeat this process several times. Always concentrate on your breathing.

D. When you explain a process, use transition words (*first, second, next, then, after that,* and *finally*). Transition words help the reader understand the order of your ideas. Circle all the transition words in the deep breathing paragraph.

What punctuation follows these transition words? ____________

Discuss the meanings of these transition words with your classmates and teacher.

E. Now, read the paragraph "Progressive Relaxation" and fill in the blanks with an appropriate transition word. There may be more than one correct answer. Use each transition word only once.

after that second finally then first next

Progressive Relaxation

Progressive relaxation is an easy way to relax your body. ____________________, sit up in your chair. Your feet should be on the floor. ____________________, close your eyes. ____________________, slowly take a deep breath (inhale). ____________________, begin with your hands and arms. Tense the muscles in your hands and your arms. Hold for five seconds. Relax your muscles. ____________________, concentrate on your chest, shoulders, and upper back. Tense the muscles in these areas. Hold for five seconds. Relax your muscles. Do the same for each of the following areas: stomach and hips, thighs, calves, and neck. Remember to breathe deeply and slowly. ____________________, open your eyes.

F. Decide on another way a person can reduce stress. Write a short paragraph for your idea. Use a clear topic sentence and correct transition words.

A Look Behind

Throughout this textbook, you studied the importance of good health. You studied the human body, medications, nutrition, exercise, and stress management. You also studied how to explain your illnesses and how to make a doctor's appointment. All of this moves you in the right direction—toward a healthier lifestyle!